Study Guide to accompany Leifer

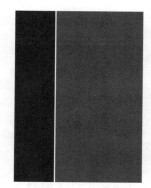

Introduction to Maternity & Pediatric Nursing

Fourth Edition

Emily Slone McKinney, MSN, RN,C
Baylor University Medical Center
Women and Children's Services
Dallas, Texas

Christine M. Rosner, RN, PhD
Assistant Professor
Division of Nursing
Holy Family College
Philadelphia, Pennsylvania

D1404145

SAUNDERS
An Imprint of Elsevier

SAUNDERS
An Imprint of Elsevier
The Curtis Center
Independence Square West
Philadelphia, Pennsylvania 19106-3399

Vice President, Publishing Director: Sally Schrefer
Senior Editor: Terri Wood
Associate Developmental Editor: Jill Riggin
Developmental Editor: Catherine Ott
Project Manager: Gayle May

Printed in the United States of America.

Last digit is the print number: 9 8 7 6 5

Preface

This Study Guide is written to promote student mastery of *Introduction to Maternity & Pediatric Nursing*, Fourth Edition, by Gloria Leifer. Each chapter in this Study Guide corresponds to the text chapter having the same number and title.

The authors have included matching and completion **Learning Activities** to help students learn basic factual knowledge that underlies nursing care. Other exercises request the student to list or describe text information to encourage reading comprehension and written expression of what is learned. Labeling of illustrations is included to help the student understand anatomy, as appropriate.

To promote higher level learning, the authors have included **Thinking Critically** activities, which ask the student to apply knowledge or draw conclusions based on material in the textbook but not directly answered in the textbook. **Case Studies** and **Applying Knowledge** activities provide ideas for applying factual content to client care.

Each chapter contains multiple choice **Review Questions**. The questions ask for appropriate nursing actions, what the nurse should expect in terms of medical orders or usual care of the client, and what complication the client is at risk of developing, as well as items that review basic factual information from the chapter. Some chapters conclude with **Crossword Puzzles** to further test comprehension of terms and concepts.

An answer key for the Learning Activities, selected Thinking Critically activities, Review Questions, and Crossword Puzzles has been provided for your instructor.

To the Student

This Study Guide was created to assist you in achieving the objectives of each chapter in *Introduction to Maternity & Pediatric Nursing*, Fourth Edition, and establishing a solid base of knowledge in maternity and pediatric nursing. Completing the exercises in each chapter in this Guide will help to reinforce the material studied in the textbook and learned in class. Such reinforcement also helps students to be successful on the NCLEX-PN.

Study Hints for All Students

Ask Questions!

There are no stupid questions. If you do not know something or are not sure, you need to find out. Other people may be wondering the same thing but may be too shy to ask. The answer could mean life or death to your patient. That is certainly more important than feeling embarrassed about asking a question.

Chapter Objectives

At the beginning of each chapter in the textbook are objectives that you should have mastered when you finish studying that chapter. Write these objectives in your notebook, leaving a blank space after each. Fill in the answers as you find them while reading the chapter. Review to make sure your answers are correct and complete. Use these answers when you study for tests. This should also be done for separate course objectives that your instructor has listed in your class syllabus.

Key Terms

At the beginning of each chapter in the textbook are key terms that you will encounter as you read the chapter. Text page number references are provided, for easy reference and review, and the key terms are in color the first time they appear in the chapter. Phonetic pronunciations are provided for terms that students might find difficult to pronounce. The terms that were assigned simple phonetic pronunciations were selected because they are either (1) difficult medical, nursing, or scientific terms or (2) other words that may be difficult for students to pronounce. The goal is to help the student reader with limited proficiency in English to develop a greater command of the pronunciation of scientific and nonscientific English terminology. It is hoped that a more general competency in the understanding and use of medical and scientific language may result.

Key Points

Use the Key Points at the end of each chapter in the textbook to help with review for exams.

Reading Hints

When reading each chapter in the textbook, look at the subject headings to learn what each section is about. Read first for the general meaning. Then reread parts you did not understand. It may help to read those parts aloud. Carefully read the information given in each table and study each figure and its caption.

Concepts

While studying, put difficult concepts into your own words to see if you understand them. Check this understanding with another student or the instructor. Write these in your notebook.

Class Notes

When taking lecture notes in class, leave a large margin on the left side of each notebook page and write only on right-hand pages, leaving all left-hand pages blank. Look over your lecture notes soon after each class, while your memory is fresh. Fill in missing words, complete sentences and ideas, and underline key phrases, definitions, and concepts. At the top of each page, write the topic of that page. In the left margin, write the key word for that part of your notes. On the opposite left-hand page, write a summary or outline that combines material from both the textbook and the lecture. These can be your study notes for review.

Study Groups

Form a study group with some other students so you can help one another. Practice speaking and reading aloud. Ask questions about material you are not sure about. Work together to find answers.

References for Improving Study Skills

Good study skills are essential for achieving your goals in nursing. Time management, efficient use of study time, and a consistent approach to studying are all beneficial. There are various study methods for reading a textbook and for taking class notes. Some methods that have proven helpful can be found in *Saunders Student Nurse Planner: A Guide to Success in Nursing School.* This book contains helpful information on test-taking and preparing for clinical experiences. It includes an example of a "time map" for planning study time and a blank form that the student can use to formulate a personal time map.

Additional Study Hints for English as a Second Language (ESL) Students

Vocabulary

If you find a nontechnical word you do not know (e.g., *drowsy*), try to guess its meaning from the sentence; e.g., *With electrolyte imbalance, the patient may feel fatigued and drowsy.* If you are not sure of the meaning, or if it seems particularly important, look it up in the dictionary.

Vocabulary Notebook

Keep a small alphabetized notebook or address book in your pocket or purse. Write down new nontechnical words you read or hear along with their meanings and pronunciations. Write each word under its initial letter so you can find it easily, as in a dictionary. For words you do not know or for words that have a different meaning in nursing, write down how they are used and sound. Look up their meanings in a dictionary or ask your instructor or first-language buddy. Then write the different meanings or usages that you have found in your book, including the nursing meaning. Continue to add new words as you discover them. For example:

primary	• of most importance; main: *the primary problem or disease*
	• the first one; elementary: *primary school*
secondary	• of less importance; resulting from another problem or disease: *a secondary symptom*
	• the second one: *secondary school (in the United States, high school)*

First-Language Buddy

ESL students should find a first-language buddy—another student who is a native speaker of English and who is willing to answer questions about word meanings, pronunciations, and culture. Maybe your buddy would like to learn about your language and culture as well. This could help in his or her nursing experience also.

Contents

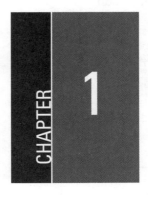

CHAPTER 1

Student Name _____

The Past, Present, and Future

Answer Key: Textbook page references are provided as a guide for answering these questions. A complete answer key was provided for your instructor.

LEARNING ACTIVITIES

1. Match the terms in the left column with their definitions on the right (a–i).

(12)	_____ advanced practice nurse	a. the difference between the expected outcome and the outcome achieved
(6)	_____ clinical pathways	b. recognizing the strength and integrity of the family as the core of planning and implementing health care
(10)	_____ diagnosis-related groups (DRG)	c. a registered nurse with an advanced degree who specializes in a clinical area of nursing such as obstetrics or pediatrics and may conduct research in their specialty
(2)	_____ empowerment	
(2)	_____ family-centered care	d. a system used by government-financed programs that determines payment for a person's hospital stay based on the diagnosis
(11)	_____ health maintenance organization (HMO)	e. a health organization that contracts with providers for services at a discount for its members
(11)	_____ managed care	f. a health care delivery system that contracts with providers to provide services at a fixed capitation fee each month
(11)	_____ preferred provider organization (PPO)	g. an organization that offers health services for a fixed premium
(6)	_____ variance	h. research-based guidelines for expected progress within a timeline
		i. providing the means by which families accept and maintain control over their members' health care

(1-2)   **2.**   List three health care professionals who deliver babies.

a. _____

b. _____

c. _____

3.   Match the names in the left column with their contributions toward improvement of maternal, newborn, and pediatric care on the right (a–j).

(2)   _____ Samuel Bard

(2)   _____ Karl Credé

(3)   _____ Abraham Jacobi

(2)   _____ Oliver Wendell Holmes

(2)   _____ Joseph Lister

(2)   _____ Louis Pasteur

(18)   _____ Margaret Sanger

(2)   _____ Ignaz Semmelweis

(2)   _____ Soranus

(3)   _____ Lillian Wald

a.   associated unwashed hands of medical students following dissection of cadavers and puerperal fever among postpartum women

b.   determined that puerperal fever was caused by bacteria that could be spread by people and objects

c.   helped establish the Children's Bureau, leading to birth registration and school lunch programs

d.   developed a treatment to prevent infant blindness caused by gonorrhea

e.   wrote a paper about the contagiousness of puerperal fever, thus initiating the germ theory of disease

f.   wrote the first American textbook on obstetrics

g.   applied antiseptic principles to surgical practice

h.   introduced podalic version to deliver the second twin

i.   established pediatric nursing as a medical specialty

j.   provided care for poor pregnant women that was the seed for development of today's Planned Parenthood programs

(3)   **4.**   List three professional organizations concerned with maternity nursing.

a. _____

b. _____

c. _____

5.   Describe how each listed governmental program influences maternity and pediatric care.

(3)   a.   Title V Amendment of the Social Security Act

_____

_____

Student Name _____

(3)   b.   Title XIX of the Medicaid program

_____

_____

(3)   c.   Head Start program

_____

_____

(3)   d.   National Center for Family Planning

_____

_____

(3)   e.   Women's, Infant's and Children's program

_____

_____

(3)   f.   Fair Labor Standards Act

_____

_____

(4)   g.   Education for All Handicapped Children Act

_____

_____

(4)   h.   Missing Children's Act

_____

_____

(6)   **6.**   How has the hospital stay for birth changed recently? What implication do you believe these changes have for nurses?

_____

_____

(7)   **7.**   How have consumers changed practices in maternity care?

_____

_____

(10)   **8.**   Give examples of how technology and development of medical specialties affects the care of infants and children.

_____

_____

_____

_____

(10)   **9.**   How have advances in technology contributed to the growing population of chronically ill children?

_____

_____

(12)   **10.**   Give two examples of advanced practice nurses.

a.   _____

b.   _____

(12-13)   **11.**   List the steps of the nursing process.

a.   _____

b.   _____

c.   _____

d.   _____

e.   _____

f.   _____

(15-16)   **12.**   Explain the meaning and use of critical thinking in nursing.

_____

_____

Student Name_____

(15)   **13.** What is the place of the Nursing Interventions Classification (NIC) and Nursing Outcome Criteria (NOC) in patient care and reimbursement for nursing services?

_____

_____

_____

_____

(17)   **14.** What is *Healthy People 2010?*

_____

_____

APPLYING KNOWLEDGE

1. What is the typical hospital stay for a woman who has an uncomplicated vaginal birth at your clinical facility? For a woman who has an uncomplicated cesarean birth? Do insurance companies or HMOs offer home visits to women who had uncomplicated births? Ask nurses how they manage their care to accommodate short postpartum hospital stays.

2. Talk with a father who was present at the birth of his child. How did the experience affect him? If he has more than one child and was not present at all the births, does he perceive any differences in how he feels toward his children based on whether he was present at their births?

3. When you are in the clinical area, care for a childbearing family from a cultural group other than your own. Use the assessment questions listed under "Cross-Cultural Considerations" in your text to better understand the family's views toward birth.

4. When you are in the clinical area, observe how the family is involved in the birth process. Talk to new grandparents about how birth has changed since their children were born. Use the following questions as a springboard to discussion or answer them alone.
    a. How do you feel about the involvement of fathers in childbirth?
    b. How do cultural influences seem to affect women and their family when birth occurs? Do you see differences between new immigrant families and those who have been in our country for more than one generation?
    c. Do you think siblings of the new baby should be involved during or after birth? If so, in what way?

5. Ask the birth facility in your clinical area what types of statistical data they gather and what is done with that data.

6. Does your clinical facility use any method of computerized charting? What security measures assure privacy of a patient's data? What arrangements does the facility have if the computer system is down?

7. List ways that you use critical thinking to solve problems or meet needs in daily non-nursing aspects of your life.

REVIEW QUESTIONS

(2) **1.** The Credé method prevents newborn eye infection by use of

1. antibiotic ointment.
2. silver nitrate solution.
3. washing each eye separately.
4. using gloves for all care.

(2) **2.** The most important nursing action to prevent infection in any patient is to

1. use disposable equipment.
2. consistently wash your hands.
3. limit visitors to family members.
4. wear hospital-laundered clothes.

(7) **3.** To best improve the care of a pregnant woman from a different cultural group, the nurse should

1. identify her expectations about pregnancy and birth.
2. observe the woman and her family as they interact.
3. learn about different local cultural groups.
4. encourage her to adopt local childbearing practices.

(7) **4.** One way in which nurses may use statistics is to

1. determine daily staffing needs in hospitals.
2. predict the hospital census for the following year.
3. evaluate the outcomes of prenatal care provided.
4. compute the number of women who conceive each year.

(15-16) **5.** Choose the care that best describes use of critical thinking in nursing care.

1. maintaining the principles of sterile technique when performing catheterization of a woman with her leg in a cast
2. assessing the likelihood of a woman being abused while her family is present

3. identifying how statistical information can be used to plan a research project
4. looking up all medications and their doses before administering them to adults and/or children

(7) **6.** Choose the best description of certified nurse-midwife (CNM) qualifications.

1. Gives limited care to women after normal childbirth.
2. Assists in the prenatal care of high-risk women.
3. Primarily provides care to low-income women.
4. Attends uncomplicated births of low-risk women.

(12-13) **7.** The nursing process is best described as a method to

1. identify patients who have an increased risk for medical complications.
2. reduce the incidence of complications for expectant mothers and infants.
3. identify and solve patient problems with individualized nursing care.
4. promote breastfeeding in groups that do not usually nurse infants.

(6) **8.** Choose the best description for a variance in a clinical pathway.

1. The patient did not cooperate with the recommended therapy.
2. An achieved patient outcome differs from the expected outcome.
3. Patient care is individualized, appropriate to a specific person.
4. Reimbursement will be curtailed because of a complication.

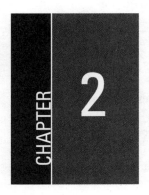

Student Name _____

CHAPTER 2

Human Reproductive Anatomy and Physiology

Answer Key: Textbook page references are provided as a guide for answering these questions. A complete answer key was provided for your instructor.

LEARNING ACTIVITIES

(21) 1. _____ is the time when reproductive systems mature and

become capable of reproduction.

(21) 2. Hormonal changes of puberty in boys begin between the ages of _____ and _____ years.

The first outward male changes of puberty are growth of the _____

and _____.

(22) 3. The first outward change of puberty in girls is _____ . The

first menstrual period usually occurs _____ after this initial

change.

(22) 4. Describe secondary sexual characteristics in boys and girls.

a. Boys _____

_____

b. Girls _____

_____

5. Match the terms in the left column with their definitions on the right (a–h).

(23) _____ androgens

(22) _____ penis

(22) _____ scrotum

(23) _____ semen

(22) _____ spermatogenesis

(23) _____ spermatozoa

(23) _____ testes

(21) _____ testosterone

a. organs that produce spermatozoa and male sex hormones
b. seminal plasma plus sperm
c. male sex hormones
d. primary male hormone
e. male germ (reproductive) cells
f. male organ for urination and sexual intercourse
g. production of spermatozoa
h. skin sac that suspends testes away from the body

(22) **6.** Label the structures of the male reproductive system on the figure below.

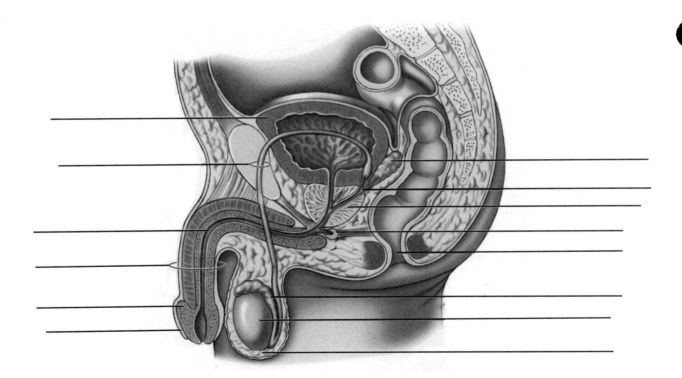

a. anus
b. bulbourethral gland
c. ejaculatory duct
d. epididymis
e. foreskin of penis

f. glans penis
g. penis
h. prostate gland
i. scrotum
j. seminal vesicle

k. testis
l. urethra
m. urinary bladder
n. vas deferens

Student Name _____

(23)   **7.**   a.   Spermatozoa are produced in the _____ of the testes.

b.   Testosterone is produced in the _____ of the testes.

(23)   **8.**   Describe six effects of testosterone.

a.   _____

b.   _____

c.   _____

d.   _____

e.   _____

f.   _____

(24)   **9.**   Label the structures of the external female genitalia on the figure below.

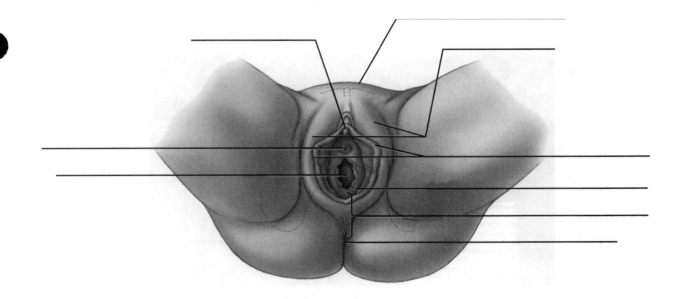

a.   anus
b.   clitoris
c.   labia majora

d.   labia minora
e.   mons pubis
f.   perineum

g.   urethra
h.   vagina

(24, 25)   **10.**   Label the structures of the internal female reproductive organs on the two figures below. Some labels are used more than once.

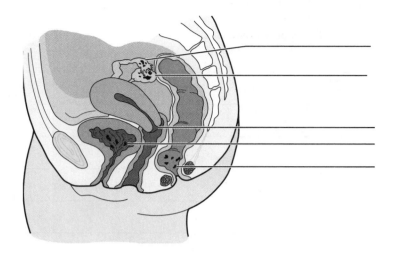

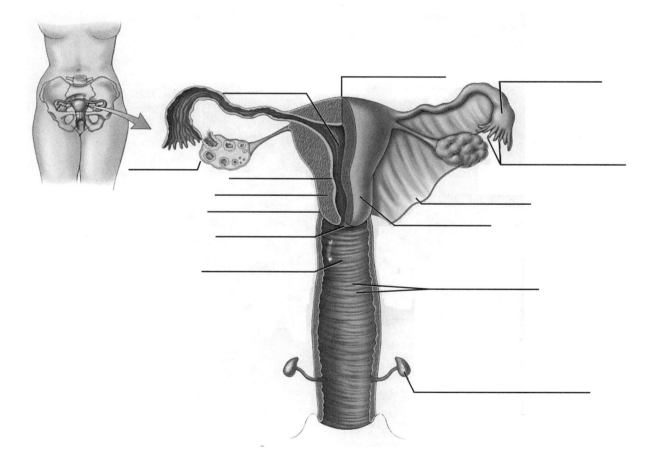

a.   bladder   d.   fallopian tube   g.   rectum

b.   broad ligament   e.   fimbriae   h.   uterine fundus

c.   cervix   f.   ovary   i.   vagina

Student Name _____

11. Match each female reproductive organ with its function or functions (a–r). More than one letter may be used for some organs.

(24) _____ Bartholin's glands (vulvovaginal glands)

(26) _____ cervical mucous membrane

(26) _____ cervix

(24) _____ clitoris

(26) _____ endometrium

(26) _____ fallopian tubes

(26) _____ myometrium

(26) _____ ovaries

(25) _____ rugae

(24) _____ Skene's ducts (paraurethral ducts)

(24) _____ urethral meatus

(25) _____ uterus

(25, 29, 31) _____ vagina

(24) _____ vaginal introitus

a. location for implantation of the fertilized ovum and growth of fetus
b. female organ of sexual intercourse
c. uterine layer that responds to hormone changes during the menstrual cycle
d. sensitive erectile body that gives erotic sensations when stimulated
e. passage for menstrual flow and fetus
f. folds or ridges of the vaginal mucous membrane
g. produce vaginal lubrication during sexual arousal
h. uterine layer in which fertilized ovum implants
i. site of fertilization and early embryonic development
j. produce ova (female germ cells) and female hormones
k. muscular uterine layer to expel fetus at birth
l. provides an environment favorable to sperm's survival
m. lubricate urethra and vaginal orifice
n. division between external and internal female genitals
o. location for urine to be expelled
p. narrow, tubular part of the uterus
q. produces the mucous plug during pregnancy
r. produces bacteriostatic vaginal lubrication

(28)   **12.** Label each diameter of the pelvic inlet on the figure below and list the normal measurements for each.

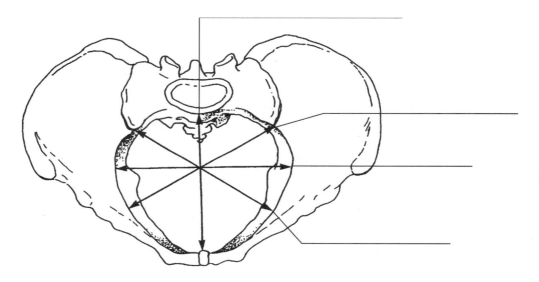

a. anteroposterior   c. left oblique   d. right oblique
b. transverse

(29)   **13.** Label each structure of the female breast on the figure below. Some labels may be used on both views.

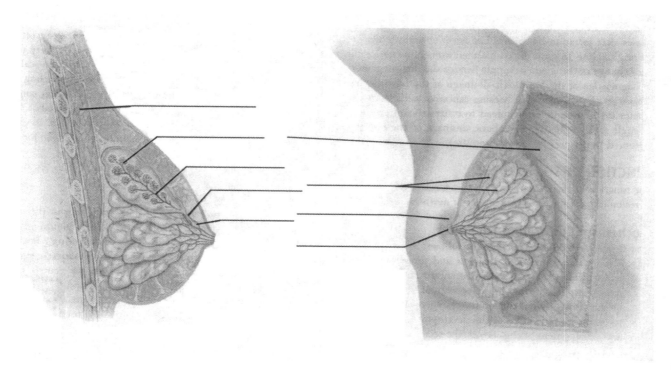

a. alveolus/alveoli   c. lactiferous duct   e. nipple
b. areola   d. lactiferous sinus   f. pectoralis major muscle

Student Name _____

● *(28-29)* **14.** Match each female breast structure with its function (a–e).

_____ alveolus/alveoli   a. widened area of a duct that holds milk

_____ areola   b. glands that secrete milk
      c. carry milk from alveoli to nipple

_____ Cooper's ligaments   d. area of darker skin surrounding nipple
      e. provide support for breast

_____ lactiferous duct

_____ lactiferous sinus

15. Match each term with its definition (a–e).

(29) _____ corpus luteum   a. painful sexual intercourse
      b. empty follicle after ovum is released

(24) _____ dyspareunia   c. first menstrual period
      d. release of mature ovum

(28) _____ follicle   e. cavity containing a single ovum

(29) _____ menarche

(29) _____ ovulation

● **16.** State where each of the following female hormones is secreted and its function or functions.

(28) a. FSH (follicle stimulating hormone)

_____

_____

(29) b. LH (luteinizing hormone)

_____

_____

(29) c. Estrogen

_____

_____

(29) d. Progesterone

● _____

_____

THINKING CRITICALLY

1.   Your 12-year-old niece confides to you that she is worried because she had her first menstrual period two months ago but has not had another one. She tells you she learned in school that most girls have periods once each month. What should you tell her?

2.   A woman is seeing the nurse practitioner because she has recurrent vaginal infections. She says she douches frequently to "keep herself clean," but that the infections often recur, especially when she needs antibiotics as she is now taking for an ear infection. What advice can the nurse give her?

APPLYING KNOWLEDGE

1.   Examine a model of the female pelvis. Identify the following landmarks.

a.   coccyx
b.   sacrum

c.   ischial spine
d.   symphysis pubis

e.   ilium
f.   linea terminalis

2.   Identify the following pelvic inlet diameters on a model of the female pelvis. Which diameter of the inlet and outlet is the shortest?

Inlet:
a.   anteroposterior
b.   left and right oblique
c.   transverse

Cavity:
a.   interspinous transverse

Outlet:
a.   anteroposterior
b.   intertuberous transverse
c.   anterior-posterior sagittal

REVIEW QUESTIONS

(22)   **1.**   The average female is usually shorter than the average male because

1.   girls have high levels of testosterone during puberty.
2.   boys begin puberty at an earlier age than girls.
3.   the growth spurt of girls ends earlier than that of boys.
4.   onset of puberty stops growth in a girl's height.

(23)   **2.**   A woman can become pregnant even if the male "pulls out" before ejaculation because

1.   ejaculation occurs before insertion of the penis.
2.   some semen is released before ejaculation.
3.   sperm are added to semen after ejaculation.
4.   semen enters the urethra as soon as the penis is inserted.

Student Name _____

(25) **3.** A woman comes to the clinic for a yearly checkup pelvic exam. She asks if it is all right for her to use a douche occasionally. The nurse should teach her that douching

   1. is unnecessary but does no harm if she prefers to do it.
   2. may hinder her vagina's natural cleansing action.
   3. adds to the natural cleansing action of her vagina.
   4. should be avoided because it makes the vagina acidic.

(26) **4.** The uterine layer that responds to hormonal changes and receives the fertilized ovum is the

   1. parametrium.
   2. myometrium.
   3. endometrium.

(27) **5.** The true pelvis is divided from the false pelvis by the

   1. obstetric conjugate.
   2. right and left oblique diameters.
   3. linea terminalis.
   4. bi-ischial diameter.

(27) **6.** The typical pelvic type for a male is the

   1. android.   2. anthropoid.
   3. gynecoid.   4. platypelloid.

(27) **7.** The ideal pelvic type for a female is the

   1. android.   2. anthropoid.
   3. gynecoid.   4. platypelloid.

(28) **8.** Which division of the female pelvis can change slightly to accommodate the fetus during birth?

   1. pelvic inlet   2. pelvic cavity
   3. pelvic outlet

(23) **9.** Males are generally stronger than females at maturity because

   1. males begin puberty at an earlier age than females.
   2. testosterone promotes growth of a male's muscles.
   3. females start puberty at a later age than males.
   4. high estrogen production promotes bone growth.

(22) **10.** The function of a male's scrotum is to

   1. regulate the temperature of the testes.
   2. carry sperm from the testes to the penis.
   3. secrete the hormone testosterone.
   4. increase the strength of ejaculation of sperm.

(28) **11.** The breast structures that secrete milk after childbirth are the

   1. lactiferous ducts.
   2. Montgomery's glands.
   3. alveoli.
   4. nipples.

(29) **12.** Erection of the penis occurs during sexual stimulation because

   1. smooth muscles attached to the pelvis lift the penis.
   2. blood is trapped within the tissues of the organ.
   3. the testosterone level falls in response to stimulation.
   4. prostate gland secretions cause the organ to stiffen.

(28)   **13.** What is the most appropriate nursing response to the woman who decides she cannot breastfeed because she has small breasts?

1. "Small breasts usually have less milk-secreting tissue, but you could give it a try when the baby arrives."
2. "Pregnancy hormones will increase most women's breast size enough to feed the average-size infant."
3. "Small breasts actually have more milk secreting glands than larger breasts; there should be plenty of milk."
4. "It is the amount of fat in your breasts that determines their size, so your chances of successfully nursing are good."

(26)   **14.** The middle layer of the myometrium has _____ fibers.

1. circular
2. figure-eight
3. longitudinal
4. oblique

(30)   **15.** The endometrium of the uterus is thinnest at what time?

1. just before ovulation
2. between ovulation and menstruation
3. at the beginning of menstruation
4. just after menstruation

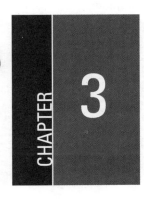

Student Name _____

CHAPTER 3

Prenatal Development

Answer Key: Textbook page references are provided as a guide for answering these questions. A complete answer key was provided for your instructor.

LEARNING ACTIVITIES

1. Match the terms in the left column with their definitions on the right (a–g).

(33)   _____ diploid

(34)   _____ gamete

(33)   _____ haploid

(33)   _____ meiosis

(33)   _____ mitosis

(33)   _____ oogenesis

(33)   _____ spermatogenesis

a. normal number of chromosomes in each mature sperm or ovum
b. normal number of chromosomes in nonreproductive cells
c. cell division in sex cells
d. cell division in nonsex cells to allow growth and replacement of cells
e. formation of spermatozoa
f. formation of ova
g. an ovum or spermatozoon

(35)   **2.** a. Spermatogenesis results in the formation of how many sperm from each immature primary spermatocyte? _____

b. Each sperm contains _____ autosomes and either a(n)

_____ or a(n) _____ sex chromosome.

(35)   **3.** a. Oogenesis results in the formation of how many mature ova from each primary oocyte?

_____

b. Each ovum contains _____ autosomes and a(n) _____ sex chromosome.

(34)   **4.**   a.   An ovum survives about _____ hours after ovulation.

b.   Sperm survive up to _____ hours after ejaculation.

(34, 37)   **5.**   a.   If the ovum is fertilized by a sperm bearing a Y chromosome, the baby will be a

_____.

b.   If the ovum is fertilized by a sperm bearing an X chromosome, the baby will be a

_____.

c.   What influence, if any, does the woman have on the sex of the baby that is conceived?

_____

_____

(34)   **6.**   Fertilization usually occurs in the _____. The

fertilized ovum usually implants in the _____ section of

the _____ uterus.

7.   Match the terms in the left column with their definitions on the right (a–j).

(36)	_____ amnion	a.	inner fetal membrane that envelops the embryo and fetus
(34)	_____ blastocyst	b.	outer fetal membrane that envelops the amnion and embryo/fetus
(34)	_____ blastomere	c.	solid cluster of cells that is approximately the same size as the zygote
(34)	_____ chorion	d.	eight-cell stage of prenatal development
(34)	_____ decidua basalis	e.	projections on the outer part of fetal side of the placenta that extend into the decidua basalis
(37)	_____ embryo	f.	prenatal development from the second week until the end of the eighth week after fertilization
(37)	_____ fetus	g.	prenatal development from the ninth week after fertilization until birth
(34)	_____ morula	h.	uterine lining after implantation that gives rise to the maternal side of the placenta
(36)	_____ chorionic villi	i.	zygote containing an inner cell mass that will develop into the embryo
(34)	_____ zygote	j.	cell formed by union of a sperm and ovum

Student Name_____

(36)   **8.**   The normal amount of amniotic fluid near the end of pregnancy is about _____ ml.

(36)   **9.**   List the five functions of amniotic fluid.

     a.   _____

     b.   _____

     c.   _____

     d.   _____

     e.   _____

(36, 42) **10.** Red blood cells are formed by the _____ for the first six

weeks after gestation and then are formed by the _____, and

finally the _____.

(37)   **11.** List the tissues that form from each of the three primary germ layers.

Ectoderm

     a.   _____

     b.   _____

     c.   _____

     d.   _____

     e.   _____

Mesoderm

     a.   _____

     b.   _____

     c.   _____

     d.   _____

     e.   _____

     f.   _____

     g.   _____

Endoderm

a. _____

b. _____

c. _____

(40)   **12.** List four functions of the placenta.

a. _____

b. _____

c. _____

d. _____

(42)   **13.** Describe the functions of each of the four following placental hormones during pregnancy.

a.   Progesterone

_____

b.   Estrogen

(1) _____

(2) _____

(3) _____

(4) _____

c.   Human chorionic gonadotropin (hCG)

_____

d.   Human placental lactogen (hPL)

_____

Student Name_____

(42-44)   **14.** Label each of the structures listed below on the drawing provided. Color areas to indicate high (red), medium (purple), and low (blue) fetal blood oxygenation. Use the lines on the neonate's illustration on the right to explain how fetal shunts close after birth.

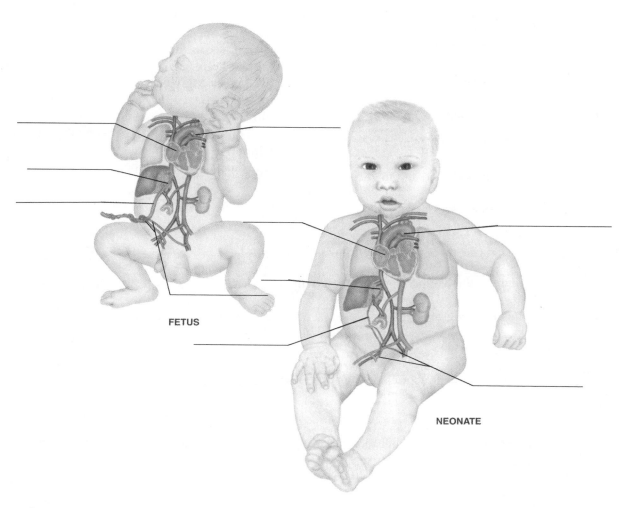

FETUS

NEONATE

a.   ductus venosus   c.   foramen ovale   e.   umbilical vein
b.   ductus arteriosus   d.   umbilical arteries

(43)   **15.** The umbilical cord should have _____ vein(s) and _____ artery(ies).

(43)   **16.** State the age when each fetal circulatory structure closes functionally and permanently.

		Functionally	**Permanently**
a.	ductus arteriosus	_____	_____
b.	ductus venosus	_____	_____
c.	foramen ovale	_____	_____

17. Match the prenatal ages with their development characteristics on the right (a–h).

(37) _____ 3 weeks

(37) _____ 6 weeks

(37) _____ 8 weeks

(37) _____ 10 weeks

(37, 40) _____ 14 weeks

(40) _____ 20 weeks

(40) _____ 28 weeks

(40) _____ 38 weeks

a. basic structure of all systems established
b. possible to monitor fetal status with kick counts
c. fetal eyes open
d. fetus now considered full term
e. tubular heart begins beating; earliest evidence of brain and spinal cord
f. external genitalia may be determined by ultrasound
g. extremities will move in response to external stimuli
h. heart has all four chambers

(42) **18.** a. Describe three things about the umbilical cord.

(1) Where it is inserted into placenta: _____

(2) Length: _____

(3) Vessels: _____

b. Explain the function of Wharton's jelly: _____

_____

(44) **19.** Describe the differences between monozygotic (identical) and dizygotic (fraternal) twins in terms of the following characteristics.

Characteristic	Monozygotic	Dizygotic
a. Same sex or different	_____	_____
b. Number of fertilized ova	_____	_____
c. Number of placentas	_____	_____
d. Number of membranes	_____	_____
e. Number of umbilical cords	_____	_____

Student Name_____

● **THINKING CRITICALLY**

1. A woman comes to the family planning clinic where you work. She wants to try a natural method of birth control rather than use artificial methods of contraception. What facts must you know about the survival time of the ovum and sperm to help your patient effectively use this form of family planning? See also Chapter 2 for information about the menstrual cycle and Chapter 11 for further information about natural family planning.

2. Your friend is disappointed because she has just had her fourth girl. "My husband wants a son so much," she says. "I feel terrible that I can't have a boy for him." What is an appropriate way to respond to your friend? Role play this situation with a classmate to refine your therapeutic communication skills.

APPLYING KNOWLEDGE

1. Examine a placenta, particularly the insertion of the umbilical cord into the placenta. Identify the following structures.
    a. amniotic membrane sac
    b. fetal side
    c. maternal side
    d. umbilical vein
    e. umbilical arteries (How do the arteries look different from the vein?)
    f. Wharton's jelly

REVIEW QUESTIONS

(37) **1.** Between the second and the eighth week of pregnancy, the developing baby is known as

1. a gamete.   2. a zygote.
3. an embryo. 4. a fetus.

(33) **2.** Cell division that results in the formation of reproductive cells is known as

1. mitosis.   2. meiosis.
3. fertilization. 4. dizygotic.

(33) **3.** How many chromosomes should be contained in the normal sperm or ovum?

1. 23   2. 46
3. 69   4. 92

(34) **4.** Which sex chromosome combination results in conception of a male?

1. XX   2. XY
3. YY   4. XO

(33) **5.** Hereditary or genetic traits are passed from one generation to the next within the

1. chromosomes.
2. zygote.
3. chorionic villi.
4. somatic cells.

(36) **6.** After six weeks gestation, fetal red blood cells are manufactured in the

1. placenta.   2. liver.
3. heart.   4. blastocyst.

(34-36)   **7.** Which is the outer fetal membrane?

1. amnion.   2. chorion.
3. syncytium.   4. vernix.

(42)   **8.** The primary function of Wharton's jelly is to

1. allow the best blood flow through the placental vessels.
2. prevent the fetal membranes from adhering to the fetal skin.
3. separate maternal blood from fetal blood in the placenta.
4. carry fetal waste products back to the placenta.

(43)   **9.** Most fetal blood bypasses circulation to the lungs by way of the

1. ductus venosus.
2. foramen ovale.
3. umbilical vein.
4. umbilical artery.

(43)   **10.** The fetal circulatory structure that carries blood with the lowest oxygen saturation is the

1. umbilical vein.
2. umbilical artery.
3. ductus venosus.
4. ductus arteriosus.

(33-34)   **11.** After fertilization, the zygote grows by

1. meiosis.   2. mitosis.
3. oogenesis.   4. gametogenesis.

(43)   **12.** The foramen ovale closes permanently in about _____ after birth.

1. 1 hour   2. 1 day
3. 3 weeks   4. 3 months

(36)   **13.** The primary purpose of amniotic fluid is to

1. speed maturation of fetal lungs.
2. prevent cold stress after birth.
3. protect the fetus during development.
4. produce hormones to maintain pregnancy.

(41)   **14.** Fetal waste products are disposed of by the

1. fetal liver.   2. placenta.
3. yolk sac.   4. endoderm.

(42)   **15.** Inadequate progesterone is likely to result in

1. release of multiple ova.
2. spontaneous abortion.
3. persistence of the corpus luteum.
4. a mixture of maternal and fetal blood.

(44)   **16.** Fraternal (dizygotic) twins result when

1. one sperm fertilizes one ovum.
2. two sperm fertilize one ovum.
3. one sperm fertilizes two ova
4. two sperm fertilize two ova.

(44)   **17.** The sex of identical (monozygotic) twins

1. is always the same.
2. may or may not be the same.
3. is always different.
4. is always one male and one female.

CHAPTER 4

Prenatal Care and Adaptations to Pregnancy

Answer Key: Textbook page references are provided as a guide for answering these questions. A complete answer key was provided for your instructor.

LEARNING ACTIVITIES

1. Match the terms in the left column with their definitions on the right (a–g).

(55)	_____ colostrum	a. breast secretion that precedes milk; rich in antibodies
(69)	_____ hemorrhoids	b. red elevations of skin with lines radiating from center
(55)	_____ mucous plug	c. varicose veins of rectum and anus
(56)	_____ pseudoanemia	d. anemia occurring because red cells increase less than plasma volume
(65)	_____ pica	e. ingestion of nonfood substances
(57)	_____ spider nevi	f. 13-week period of pregnancy
(51)	_____ trimester	g. seals cervical canal during pregnancy

2. Match the terms describing a woman's obstetrical history with their definitions on the right (a–h).

(50)	_____ abortion	a. pregnancy, regardless of duration; pregnant woman
(50)	_____ gravida	b. woman pregnant for the first time
(50)	_____ multigravida	c. woman pregnant for the second or subsequent time
(50)	_____ multipara	d. woman who has not delivered a pregnancy of at least 20 weeks gestation
(50)	_____ nullipara	e. woman who delivered one or more pregnancies after at least 20 weeks gestation
(50)	_____ para	f. woman who has delivered one pregnancy of at least 20 weeks gestation
(50)	_____ primigravida	g. woman who has delivered two or more pregnancies of at least 20 weeks gestation
(50)	_____ primipara	h. end of pregnancy before 20 weeks of gestation

(51)   **3.**   _____ is a formula used to

calculate a woman's estimated date of delivery (EDD). Describe how to use this formula.

_____

_____

_____

(52-53)   **4.**   Describe the presumptive signs of pregnancy.

a.   _____

b.   _____

c.   _____

d.   _____

e.   _____

f.   _____

g.   _____

These signs and symptoms are called *presumptive* because _____

_____ .

(53-54)   **5.**   Describe the probable signs of pregnancy.

a.   _____

b.   _____

c.   _____

d.   _____

e.   _____

f.   _____

g.   _____

h.   _____

i.   _____

j.   _____

Student Name_____

These signs and symptoms are called *probable* because _____

_____

_____

(54) **6.** Describe positive signs of pregnancy. At what time during pregnancy can each be detected?

a. _____

_____

b. _____

_____

c. _____

_____

7. Match the signs and symptoms of pregnancy with their descriptions on the right (a–l).

(53) _____ abdominal striae

(51) _____ amenorrhea

(53) _____ ballottement

(53) _____ Braxton Hicks contractions

(53) _____ Chadwick's sign

(52) _____ chloasma gravidarum

(54) _____ funic souffle

(53) _____ Goodell's sign

(53) _____ Hegar's sign

(52) _____ linea nigra

(52) _____ quickening

(54) _____ uterine souffle

a. bluish color of cervix, vagina, and vulva
b. stretch marks
c. rebound of fetal part when tapped by examining finger during vaginal examination
d. softened lower uterus
e. irregular, painless uterine contractions
f. blowing sound heard over uterus
g. swishing sound of blood circulating through umbilical cord
h. cessation of menses
i. softened cervix and vagina
j. darker pigmented line in midline of abdomen
k. movement of fetus felt by mother
l. brownish pigmentation of face ("mask of pregnancy")

(54)   **8.**   a.   _____ is the hormone detected in a

positive pregnancy test.

      b.   Two body fluids used for pregnancy tests are _____

and _____.

(53-55)   **9.**   Describe changes that occur in the reproductive organs during pregnancy.

      a.   Uterus

Size _____

Weight _____

Capacity _____

      b.   Cervix_____

_____

      c.   Ovaries _____

_____

      d.   Vagina _____

_____

   10.   Describe changes in other body systems during pregnancy.

(55)   a.   Breasts _____

_____

(55)   b.   Respiratory_____

_____

_____

(55-56)   c.   Cardiovascular _____

_____

_____

_____

Student Name_____

(56-57)   d.   Gastrointestinal _____

_____

_____

_____

(57)   e.   Urinary_____

_____

_____

_____

(57-58)   f.   Integumentary and skeletal _____

_____

_____

_____

(60)   **11.**   Describe the recommended weight gain if the woman's prepregnancy weight is as follows:

a.   Normal: _____ to _____ pounds (_____ to _____ kg)

b.   Underweight: _____ to _____ pounds (_____ to _____ kg)

c.   Overweight: _____ to _____ pounds (_____ to _____ kg)

(60, 65)   **12.**   The recommended calorie increase during pregnancy is _____ calories per day.

During lactation, the recommended calorie increase is _____ calories per day.

(61)   **13.**   For the following four nutrients, state the amount needed during pregnancy for an adult and list key food sources for each nutrient. Practice how you would actually teach the information to a pregnant woman.

a.   Protein

Amount _____

Sources _____

_____

_____

b.   Calcium

Amount _____

Sources _____

_____

_____

c.   Iron

Amount _____

Sources _____

_____

_____

d.   Folic acid

Amount _____

Sources _____

_____

_____

14.   Describe how the nurse can help women meet special nutritional needs during pregnancy.

(64)   a.   Pregnant adolescent

_____

_____

_____

(61, 65)   b.   Lactose intolerance

_____

_____

_____

Student Name_____

(68-70)   **15.** List at least three measures the nurse can teach a woman to relieve each common pregnancy discomfort. Note any related abnormal signs or symptoms that should be reported. Practice explaining each relief measure to a pregnant woman.

a. Nausea

_____

_____

_____

b. Increased vaginal discharge

_____

_____

_____

c. Fatigue

_____

_____

_____

d. Backache

_____

_____

_____

e. Constipation

_____

_____

_____

f. Varicose veins

_____

_____

_____

g.   Hemorrhoids

_____

_____

_____

h.   Heartburn

_____

_____

_____

i.   Dyspnea and nasal stuffiness

_____

_____

_____

j.   Leg cramps

_____

_____

_____

k.   Edema of the legs

_____

_____

_____

(70-72)   **16.** Describe the common emotional reactions of a woman during each trimester of pregnancy.

a.   First _____

_____

b.   Second _____

_____

Student Name _____

    c.   Third _____

_____

_____

THINKING CRITICALLY

1. Today is June 19. A woman is admitted to the hospital in labor. She tells you that her "due date" is June 26. How many weeks pregnant is the woman?

2. If a woman's expected date of delivery is July 21, what was the first day of her last menstrual period?

3. Have a discussion group that contains both men and women who have had children (they do not have to be nurses or nursing students). Discuss the parts fathers played in any births. Explore the feelings of men in the group about how they view their role in childbirth.

CASE STUDIES

1. Rosa Garza comes to the clinic for a regular visit at 26 weeks gestation. Her weight gain has been normal (17 pounds), but Rosa tells you that her mother cautioned her not to gain more than 20 pounds or it will be hard to lose the weight after she gives birth. "My mother said that I should not eat salt and that the doctor will probably give me 'water pills' if I gain too much weight." What teaching should you give Rosa about each of her concerns?
   a. Weight gain
   b. Salt (sodium) intake
   c. Diuretics (water pills)

2. Lauren Holt, 30 years old, is pregnant for the first time. She describes herself as a vegetarian, although she says she occasionally eats dairy products and eggs. What nutritional advice can the nurse provide, considering Lauren's pregnancy needs and her food preferences?

APPLYING KNOWLEDGE

1. Each date below represents the first day of a woman's last menstrual period. Use a wheel to calculate the expected date of delivery for each. If you have access to an electronic gestation calculator, use it to make the same calculations. Using today's date, figure how many weeks the pregnancy has advanced.
   a. January 18
   b. July 13
   c. December 30

2. Use the TPALM system to describe each of the following pregnancy histories.
   a. A woman is pregnant for the fourth time. She had one spontaneous abortion, one child born at 32 weeks gestation who is living, and another living child born at 41 weeks gestation.
   b. A woman is 32 weeks pregnant with her second pregnancy. Her first pregnancy ended with a spontaneous abortion at 8 weeks gestation.

REVIEW QUESTIONS

(52) **1.** When a woman is 20 weeks pregnant, she is expected to experience

1. nausea and vomiting.
2. movement of the fetus.
3. burning during urination.
4. yellowish vaginal discharge.

(70-72) **2.** A woman is 18 weeks pregnant. During a prenatal visit, she tells the nurse she is worried that her baby might not be normal. How should the nurse interpret this statement?

1. Concerns about fetal well-being are common during early pregnancy.
2. It is unusual for women to have these feelings because they do not perceive the baby as "real."
3. She may have underlying rejection of the fetus that is being expressed in this way.
4. Her image of the fetus is not realistic, so the nurse should not be concerned.

(70-72) **3.** A woman's emotional reaction during the second trimester of pregnancy may be characterized by

1. fear for her safety during labor.
2. passive and dependent behavior.
3. fantasies about the baby's appearance.
4. dramatic changes in her moods.

(55) **4.** The purpose of the mucous plug is to

1. increase the blood supply to the uterus.
2. block ascent of infection to the uterus.
3. soften and stretch the cervix.
4. lubricate the vaginal walls.

(55) **5.** While lying on the examining table during her prenatal check, a woman complains of being dizzy and weak. She is pale and her skin is moist. The best nursing intervention to relieve her symptoms is to

1. have her turn to her side.
2. tell her to take deep breaths.
3. help her sit up on the table.
4. elevate her feet and legs.

(60) **6.** A woman who is underweight at the beginning of pregnancy should gain how much weight during pregnancy?

1. 15–25 pounds
2. 25–35 pounds
3. 28–40 pounds
4. more than 40 pounds

Student Name _____

(61) 7. To ensure that a woman has adequate iron intake during pregnancy, it is often recommended that she

1. drink at least one quart of milk per day.
2. take 30 mg of an iron supplement daily.
3. eat combinations of meat and grains.
4. eat 18 mg of iron daily in a variety of foods.

(69) 8. What should the nurse teach a pregnant woman about caring for varicose veins in her legs?

1. Apply warm packs to the legs.
2. Sit down as much as possible.
3. Stretch the legs while pointing toes.
4. Elevate the legs when sitting.

(47) 9. The primary goal of prenatal care is to assure the woman of

1. labor with a minimum of pain.
2. the healthiest outcome possible.
3. improved long-term nutrition.
4. minimal pregnancy discomforts.

(50) 10. A woman who is pregnant with her first baby is called a

1. multigravida.
2. para.
3. nullipara.
4. primipara.

(61) 11. Which of these foods are the highest in iron?

1. citrus fruits and melons
2. milk, cheese, and other dairy products
3. dried beans, potatoes, and legumes
4. meat and dark green vegetables

(61) 12. Adequate stores of folic acid are needed before conception to

1. promote adequate expansion of the blood volume.
2. reduce nausea and vomiting in the first trimester.
3. limit depletion of calcium from the mother's teeth.
4. reduce the risk for fetal neural tube defects.

(60) 13. The end outcome (goal) for the nursing diagnosis Altered nutrition: Less than body requirements related to low prepregnancy weight, is that the patient will

1. identify recommended nutrient intake during pregnancy.
2. gain at least 28 pounds by the end of pregnancy.
3. recognize that good nutrition promotes maternal and fetal health.
4. state the appropriate calorie increase for pregnancy.

(51) 14. The first day of a woman's last menstrual period was September 5. Her estimated date of delivery (EDD) is

1. April 12.   2. May 5.
3. June 12.   4. July 16.

(68-69) 15. Choose the most appropriate teaching for the nursing diagnosis of Constipation related to effects of pregnancy.

1. Take a mild laxative no more than three times per week.
2. Eat several servings of raw fruits and vegetables each day.
3. Limit fluids to one quart each day, taken between meals.
4. Wait until the environment is quiet before defecating.

(69)   **16.** The expectant mother is more likely to have leg cramps if she

1. does not take her iron supplement each day.
2. increases her fluid intake to eight glasses per day.
3. stretches each leg while flexing the foot three times each day.
4. drinks at least 1 to 1.5 quarts of milk each day.

(68)   **17.** A pregnant woman calls the prenatal clinic and says she has a profuse yellow vaginal discharge. The nurse should instruct the woman to

1. douche with a commercial vinegar and water solution.
2. avoid sexual intercourse until the symptoms go away.
3. wear cotton panties that allow adequate air circulation.
4. come to the clinic for further evaluation by the physician.

(68)   **18.** The most appropriate teaching for relief of nausea during early pregnancy is to

1. divide daily food intake into several small meals.
2. sit upright for 30–60 minutes after meals.
3. drink at least 8 ounces of liquid with each meal.
4. eat dry toast or crackers each night before sleep.

(52)   **19.** A pregnant woman is concerned about the "ugly brown spots" on her face. The nurse should teach her that

1. unscented skin lotions may reduce the darkness of the areas.
2. these are temporary changes due to increased hormones.
3. she should avoid wearing makeup until the areas fade.
4. iron supplements sometimes cause temporary skin darkening.

(57)   **20.** It is important to maintain adequate fluid intake during pregnancy primarily to prevent

1. orthostatic hypotension.
2. edema of the feet and legs.
3. nausea and vomiting.
4. urinary tract infection.

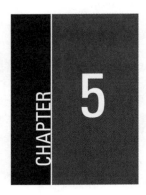

Student Name _____

Nursing Care of Women with Complications During Pregnancy

Answer Key: Textbook page references are provided as a guide for answering these questions. A complete answer key was provided for your instructor.

LEARNING ACTIVITIES

1. Match the terms in the left column with their definitions on the right (a–f).

(93) _____ abruptio placentae

(86) _____ ectopic pregnancy

(81) _____ hyperemesis gravidarum

(84) _____ incompetent cervix

(91) _____ placenta previa

(84, 86) _____ spontaneous abortion

a. placental attachment in the lower uterus
b. premature separation of the normally implanted placenta
c. spontaneous loss of a pregnancy before 20 weeks (often called *miscarriage*)
d. failure of the cervix to remain closed until the fetus is mature enough to survive outside the uterus
e. excessive nausea and vomiting during pregnancy
f. development of the fetus outside the uterus

(84) 2. List four or more appropriate nursing interventions for the woman with hyperemesis gravidarum.

a. _____

_____

b. _____

_____

c. _____

_____

d. _____

_____

(86)   **3.**   Match the types of spontaneous abortion with their descriptions on the right (a–h).

_____ threatened

_____ incomplete

_____ inevitable

_____ complete

_____ missed

_____ recurrent

_____ therapeutic

_____ elective

a.   bleeding and cramping with cervical dilation but no passage of tissue

b.   bleeding and cramping with passage of some tissue

c.   intentional termination of pregnancy for health reasons

d.   intentional termination of pregnancy for reasons unrelated to health

e.   passage of all products of conception

f.   retention of the dead fetus in the uterus

g.   two or more consecutive spontaneous abortions (also called *habitual abortion*)

h.   vaginal bleeding without dilation of the cervix or passage of tissue

(85)   **4.**   Describe important teaching for a woman after spontaneous abortion for each aspect listed.

a.   Bleeding _____

_____

b.   Temperature _____

_____

c.   Iron supplementation _____

_____

d.   Resuming sexual activity _____

_____

e.   Contraception _____

_____

(86)   **5.**   An ectopic pregnancy usually occurs in the _____

_____.

(90)   **6.**   The priority nursing observation related to ectopic pregnancy is for

_____.

Student Name _____

(90-91) **7.** Describe each characteristic of gestational trophoblastic disease that manifests as hydatidiform mole.

    a.   Bleeding _____

            _____

    b.   Uterine size _____

            _____

    c.   Fetal heart activity _____

            _____

    d.   Presence of vomiting _____

            _____

    e.   Blood pressure _____

            _____

    f.   Human chorionic gonadotropin (hCG) levels _____

            _____

    g.   Ultrasound appearance _____

            _____

    h.   Risk for cancer _____

            _____

(92) **8.** Describe the location of each type of placenta previa.

    a.   Marginal _____

            _____

    b.   Partial _____

            _____

    c.   Total _____

            _____

(91-93) **9.** How does placenta previa compare to abruptio placentae in each of the following characteristics?

	Placenta Previa	**Abruptio Placentae**
Pain		
Characteristics of bleeding		
Fetal anemia and/or hypoxia		
Consistency of the uterus		
Blood coagulation		
Risk for postpartum hemorrhage		
Risk for postpartum infection		

Student Name _____

(81, 95)   **10.**   Using Box 5-1, Danger Signs in Pregnancy, choose the factors that suggest development of pregnancy-induced hypertension and the cause of each. Which of these suggest that a seizure may occur soon if there is no intervention?

_____

_____

_____

_____

_____

_____

_____

_____

(94)   **11.**   List six or more factors that increase a woman's risk for development of pregnancy-induced hypertension (PIH).

a.   _____

b.   _____

c.   _____

d.   _____

e.   _____

f.   _____

(94)   **12.**   Describe each variation of pregnancy-induced hypertension.

a.   Pregnancy-induced hypertension _____

_____

b.   Preeclampsia _____

_____

c.   Eclampsia _____

_____

d.   HELLP _____

_____

e.   Chronic hypertension _____

_____

f.   Transient gestational hypertension _____

_____

(95)   **13.**   What blood pressure elevation is significant during pregnancy? _____

_____

(94-95)   **14.**   Describe manifestations of preeclampsia and the cause of each. Note those that suggest severe preeclampsia.

a.   Hypertension _____

_____

b.   Edema _____

_____

c.   Proteinuria _____

_____

d.   Central nervous system changes _____

_____

e.   Visual disturbances _____

_____

f.   Urine output _____

_____

g.   Pulmonary edema _____

_____

h.   Epigastric pain (upper abdominal, over stomach) or nausea _____

_____

_____

i.   Lab study abnormalities (liver enzymes, coagulation) _____

_____

Student Name _____

● *(96)* **15.** What is the benefit of activity restriction in treatment of preeclampsia? _____

_____

(96-97) **16.** a. What is the purpose of magnesium sulfate in the treatment of PIH?

_____

b. What observations are needed for a woman who is receiving magnesium sulfate as treatment for hypertension?

_____

c. What drug should be on hand if a woman is receiving magnesium sulfate?

_____

d. What is the desired serum level of magnesium when treating a woman with preeclampsia?

_____

● *(99)* **17.** a. Rh blood incompatibility can only occur if the mother is Rh _____

and the fetus is Rh _____.

(100) b. The drug given to prevent Rh incompatibility is _____

_____.

(100) c. List four instances in which the drug listed in part (b) is indicated.

(1) _____

(2) _____

(3) _____

(4) _____

(100) **18.** a. ABO incompatibility is more likely to occur in which maternal blood group or groups?

_____

b. In which fetal blood group or groups? _____

● *(100)* **19.** Which type of diabetes occurs only during pregnancy? _____

(102)   **20.** Describe the test used to screen for gestational diabetes and the normal results. When is screening done?

_____

_____

_____

(102)   **21.** a.   Why is glucose monitored by blood testing during pregnancy?

_____

_____

b.   What place does urine testing have in diabetes management during pregnancy?

_____

(102)   **23.** The preferred drug used to control the blood glucose during pregnancy is _____

_____ because it

_____.

(102)   **24.** Describe how insulin requirements change during the course of pregnancy and after birth.

_____

_____

(102, 105) **25.** How may exercise needs differ in the woman who has preexisting diabetes and the woman with gestational diabetes?

_____

_____

_____

(106)   **26.** How may the normal changes of pregnancy affect the woman with heart disease?

_____

_____

_____

Student Name _____

(106) **27.** How do labor and the postpartum period change the demands on the heart?

_____

_____

(107) **28.** List three reasons why a pregnant woman needs increased iron.

    a. _____

    b. _____

    c. _____

(107) **29.** A hemoglobin level lower than _____ g/dl indicates anemia during pregnancy.

(108) **30.** List foods high in the following nutrients.

    a. Iron _____

_____

_____

    b. Folic acid _____

_____

_____

    c. Vitamin C_____

_____

_____

(108) **31.** a. What types of foods are good to take with an iron supplement and why?

_____

      b. What foods or drugs should be avoided at the time an iron supplement is taken and why?

_____

_____

(107) **32.** What are the differences in supplementation of folic acid for routine prevention and actual folic acid deficiency? What two conditions may adequate folic acid intake prevent?

_____

(108)   **33.**   What is the effect of a sickle cell crisis during pregnancy? _____

_____

34.   Match each infection with the method to prevent infection of the fetus or newborn on the right (a–f).

(109)   _____ cytomegalovirus

(109)   _____ rubella

(109)   _____ herpesvirus

(109)   _____ hepatitis B

(110)   _____ toxoplasmosis

(111)   _____ group B streptococcus

a.   deliver infant by cesarean birth if the woman has genital lesions when labor begins

b.   give immune globulin immediately after birth followed by vaccine

c.   immunize children to avoid infecting pregnant women; immunize nonimmune woman after birth

d.   treat culture-positive woman and her infant with penicillin

e.   wash hands and surfaces after handling raw meat, cook meat thoroughly, avoid cat litter

f.   no effective prevention or treatment

(109)   **35.**   What are the recommendations to prevent hepatitis B in the newborn?

_____

_____

(110)   **36.**   List three ways an infant may be infected with human immunodeficiency virus (HIV).

a.   _____

b.   _____

c.   _____

(110)   **37.**   What teaching about the following is appropriate to prevent the spread of AIDS?

a.   Drug abuse _____

b.   Sexual intercourse _____

(112)   **38.**   Why is a pregnant woman more likely to have a urinary tract infection?

_____

_____

(112)   **39.**   List at least three things the nurse can teach a woman about avoiding a urinary tract infection.

a.   _____

_____

Student Name _____

b. _____

_____

c. _____

_____

(113) **40.** Describe general approaches to the care of pregnant women related to bioterrorist attacks.

_____

_____

_____

(114) **41. a.** Describe the manifestations of fetal alcohol syndrome (FAS).

_____

_____

_____

b. What is the current recommendation about alcohol intake during pregnancy?

_____

_____

(114-115) **42.** Match each substance with its potential adverse effects when used during pregnancy or appropriate preventive measures (a–i).

_____ ACE inhibitors	a.	abstinence syndrome may develop in woman or infant if drug is stopped suddenly
_____ cigarette smoking	b.	associated with congenital heart disease and toxicity to fetal thyroid and kidneys
_____ cocaine	c.	causes spontaneous abortion and other serious fetal anomalies
_____ folic acid antagonists	d.	crosses placenta, possibly causing spontaneous abortion, growth restriction, and central nervous system and facial defects
_____ heroin	e.	fetal kidney abnormalities, growth restriction, and insufficient amniotic fluid
_____ lithium	f.	infant may be smaller than expected for gestation
_____ tetracycline	g.	infant may have discolored teeth
_____ vitamin A preparations (isotretinoin [Accutane])	h.	reliable birth control is needed for three months after treatment with this drug
_____ warfarin	i.	severe vasoconstriction may cause preterm labor, hypertension with reduced placental circulation, and maternal stroke

(114)   **43.**   If a woman needs a potentially teratogenic therapeutic drug during pregnancy, how will the health care provider make a decision about what to prescribe?

_____

_____

(116)   **44.**   What are the risks to a woman and her infant if she is a victim of abuse?

_____

_____

_____

(116)   **45.**   List manifestations of battering.

_____

_____

_____

_____

THINKING CRITICALLY

1.   How might anemia affect a woman who has heart disease?

2.   You are helping to care for a woman receiving intravenous magnesium sulfate. You note that her urine output has decreased, and was 20 ml during the past hour. What is the significance of your observation? What is the appropriate action? Why?

3.   When a couple loses a baby because of spontaneous abortion, how do you think their friends and family are likely to react? What emotional support is appropriate if the woman believes that she should not feel sad because she did not really know the baby yet? How can the nurse help the family cope with this crisis? (These questions can also be enacted by a small group and show both therapeutic and nontherapeutic responses by the nurse.)

CASE STUDY

1.   a.   Amy Adams, 28 years old, is pregnant for the fifth time. She has had two spontaneous abortions and one stillborn baby who was born at 35 weeks of gestation. Amy's only living child, Sam, weighed 10 pounds, 3 ounces when born at 36 weeks gestation. Amy had hypertension in her pregnancy with Sam and with her stillborn baby. She is at the clinic for a routine prenatal check at 12 weeks. Her weight gain is normal, but she began pregnancy about 25 pounds overweight. All other prenatal checks are normal.

Student Name _____

Identify three or more factors that predispose Amy to complications in this pregnancy. Can any of the risk factors be modified safely? What prenatal assessments may identify these complications early? What danger signals in pregnancy should you teach Amy?

b.   Amy's pregnancy progresses normally until 28 weeks gestation. Both the glucose screen (glucose challenge test) and a glucose tolerance test were abnormal, and Amy must take insulin injections twice a day to control her gestational diabetes. What teaching will Amy need for this new problem?

c.   Amy is 35 weeks pregnant. Her gestational diabetes has been well-controlled, although she has needed higher doses of insulin as pregnancy progressed. She has now developed mild preeclampsia, and her physician advises her to remain on bed rest at home. What teaching is important about Amy's therapy for preeclampsia? How can the nurse help Amy and her family cope with the stresses of her high-risk pregnancy?

APPLYING KNOWLEDGE

1.   Assist the experienced nurse in assessing each of these reflexes. Will any of these be inaccurate when a woman has epidural analgesia or anesthesia for birth?
     a.   patellar
     b.   biceps
     c.   triceps

2.   Study your hospital's policies and procedures for nursing care related to magnesium sulfate therapy for preeclampsia or eclampsia.

3.   Observe the nursing care of a woman who is receiving magnesium sulfate for PIH. What is the reason for each nursing intervention specifically related to magnesium sulfate administration? Did the woman have any of the risk factors for PIH listed in Box 5-3 in the textbook?

REVIEW QUESTIONS

(101) **1.** A pregnant woman with insulin-dependent diabetes mellitus asks the nurse why she has needed several increases in her insulin dose during pregnancy. The best answer is that the

1. changes of pregnancy decrease the secretion of insulin from the pancreas.
2. placenta secretes substances that decrease the effectiveness of insulin.
3. fetus does not yet secrete insulin and needs more from the mother.
4. pancreas secretes progressively less insulin as pregnancy progresses.

(97) **2.** During a seizure, the priority nursing action for the pregnant woman is to

1. maintain the woman's safety to prevent injury.
2. provide supplemental oxygen by face mask.
3. insert something between her teeth.
4. give an anticonvulsant medication.

(83) **3.** The purpose of the biophysical profile (BPP) is to

1. assess the amount of blood incompatibility between the mother and fetus.
2. determine if the fetal lungs are mature enough to survive extrauterine life.
3. determine if the placenta is functioning well enough to support fetal life.
4. identify serious congenital abnormalities during early pregnancy.

(109) **4.** If a pregnant woman is not immune to rubella, the expected action is to

1. limit her contact with other pregnant women.
2. immunize her early in the postpartum period.
3. inform her that her baby may have defects.
4. tell her that there is little risk for problems.

(112) **5.** Select the most appropriate teaching for the woman who is prone to urinary tract infections.

1. Wipe the perineal area in a front-to-back direction.
2. Eat a diet high in fiber, iron, and vitamin C.
3. Eat a diet that includes additional citrus fruits and drinks.
4. Avoid using added lubricant during sexual intercourse.

(106) **6.** If a woman has cardiac disease, the main risks to the fetus are related to

1. poor oxygenation.
2. preterm birth.
3. maternal infection.
4. congenital anomalies.

(81) **7.** Which of the following fetal or neonatal problems should the nurse anticipate if a woman has persistent hyperemesis gravidarum?

1. multiple vitamin and mineral deficiencies
2. poor attachment behaviors at birth
3. smaller than expected birth weight
4. intrauterine infection or neonatal sepsis

Student Name _____

(85, 90) **8.** Choose the maternal sign or symptom that is most characteristic of hypovolemic shock associated with blood loss in a pregnant woman.

1. oral temperature below 36.1° C (97° F)
2. abnormal uterine contractions
3. urine output of 100 ml/hour
4. weak pulse that increases in rate

(89) **9.** Choose the assessment that should be promptly reported to the physician when a woman is being observed in the emergency room for possible ectopic pregnancy.

1. pulse of 88 and blood pressure of 124/66
2. light vaginal bleeding without cramping
3. oral temperature of 37.3° C (99.2° F)
4. fall in urine output to 20 ml/hour

(90) **10.** The nurse should emphasize the importance of long-term follow-up care for the woman who has a hydatidiform mole to detect the occurrence of

1. recurrent pregnancy.
2. choriocarcinoma.
3. hypertension.
4. continued bleeding.

(92) **11.** A significant difference between the signs of abruptio placentae and those of placenta previa is that abruptio placentae involves

1. bleeding. 2. infection.
3. vomiting. 4. pain.

(91, 93) **12.** A woman is admitted to the hospital with painless vaginal bleeding at 36 weeks of gestation. Which test should the nurse expect?

1. x-ray
2. ultrasound
3. vaginal exam
4. alpha-fetoprotein

(94) **13.** The cause of preeclampsia is

1. poor nutrition.
2. excess weight gain.
3. multiple fetuses.
4. unknown.

(94-95) **14.** A woman who is hospitalized with severe preeclampsia should be closely observed for the onset of

1. seizures.
2. proteinuria.
3. hypotension.
4. edema.

(96) **15.** The drug used to reverse magnesium toxicity is

1. ferrous oxide.
2. calcium gluconate.
3. Ringer's lactate.
4. magnesium chloride.

(109) **16.** Teaching of the woman who has herpesvirus infection should include

1. antibiotic treatment of the baby after birth.
2. the possibility of birth by cesarean delivery.
3. the minor effects of herpes infection on a newborn.
4. that immunity is permanent after initial infection.

(111) **17.** The physician wants to do a group B streptococcus culture when a woman has a prenatal visit at 35 weeks gestation. The woman asks the nurse why the physician is just now concerned about this problem. The best explanation by the nurse is that

1. determining if she is positive for the organism reduces the risk for spreading it by unwashed or inadequately washed hands.
2. the woman can carry the organism without knowing it, possibly causing serious infections to her or the newborn.
3. late-pregnancy infection causes significant delay in fetal lung maturation, causing problems similar to those of prematurity.
4. tissues of the vaginal and perineal area are more susceptible to tearing at birth when infection occurs during late pregnancy.

(102) **18.** The nurse should expect to teach the pregnant woman with gestational diabetes to monitor her glucose by

1. assessing blood levels several times a day.
2. determining levels in the urine twice a day.
3. recording monthly glycosylated hemoglobin levels.
4. keeping a written record of hypoglycemic symptoms.

(111) **19.** Teaching for the pregnant woman who was newly diagnosed with tuberculosis should include

1. increasing fluid intake to 2 quarts each day.
2. the expectation that birth will require a cesarean delivery.
3. the importance of taking the entire course of medication.
4. avoiding contact with family members until all medication is taken.

(116) **20.** To improve circulation to the placenta in a pregnant woman who has been in a serious car accident, the nurse should

1. place the woman in a slight head-down position on any bed or examining table.
2. give all intravenous fluids by pump to reduce fluid overload on her heart.
3. take vital signs every 15 minutes if her condition is not stable.
4. place a small pillow under one hip if she must lie on her back.

CHAPTER 6

Student Name _____

6 Nursing Care During Labor and Birth

Answer Key: Textbook page references are provided as a guide for answering these questions. A complete answer key was provided for your instructor.

LEARNING ACTIVITIES

(124) **1.** List the "4 Ps" of the birth process.

a. _____

b. _____

c. _____

d. _____

(124) **2.** The two powers of labor are:

a. _____

b. _____

(124) **3.** a. The amount of cervical dilation is expressed in _____.

b. Cervical effacement is expressed as _____

_____ .

(124-125) **4.** The nurse should promptly report contraction durations longer than _____ seconds or intervals shorter than _____ seconds and a frequency closer than every _____ minutes. Why?

_____

_____

_____

_____

(127)   **5.**   State two reasons why the sutures and fontanels of the fetal head are important the birth process.

  a.   _____

  _____

  b.   _____

  _____

(128, 130) **6.**   The abbreviations below describe fetal presentation and position. Spell out each and identify the one describing a breech presentation, the one describing a face presentation, and the one that is the most common of those listed. Identify the abbreviation that often causes "back labor" during birth.

  a.   RSA _____

  b.   LMT _____

  c.   ROA _____

  d.   LOP _____

(135, 136) **7.**   The key difference between true labor and false labor is _____

  _____.

(144, 145) **8.**   List the three phases of the first stage of labor. Describe cervical changes and the approximate duration of each phase.

  a.   _____

  _____

  b.   _____

  _____

  c.   _____

  _____

(146, 148) **9.**   The fourth stage of labor is _____.

Student Name _____

(145-146) **10.** Describe typical maternal behaviors or occurrences during each stage and phase of labor.

    a.   First stage

        Latent phase _____

        _____

        Active phase _____

        _____

        Transition phase _____

        _____

    b.   Second stage _____

        _____

    c.   Third stage _____

        _____

    d.   Fourth stage _____

        _____

(136, 137) **11.** Describe characteristics of the normal fetal heart rate at term.

    Rate _____ (lower limit) to _____ (upper limit)

    Other characteristics _____

    _____

(141) **12.** Describe three characteristics of abnormal amniotic fluid.

    _____

    _____

(140-141) **13.** Describe the assessments in the following categories that the nurse should promptly report when caring for a laboring woman.

    a.   Temperature _____

    b.   Blood pressure _____

    c.   Fetal heart rate _____

    _____

(137-141) **14.** What is the significance of the following patterns on the electronic fetal monitor? Include the nursing response to each, as appropriate.

    a.   Variability _____

            _____

            _____

    b.   Accelerations _____

            _____

    c.   Early decelerations _____

            _____

    d.   Variable decelerations _____

            _____

    e.   Late decelerations _____

            _____

THINKING CRITICALLY

1. The following chart shows a typical status report often used in intrapartum units. Interpret the data about each woman's labor by answering the questions below.

Name	Gravida	Para	Gest	Dil	Eff	Sta	FHR
Amy	2	0	36	1–2	50%	–2	160
Becky	4	3	42	6	80%	–1	115
Cathy	1	0	40	3–4	90%	0	144
Deanna	3	1	39	C	C	+2	132

    a.   Which client(s) is/are at full-term gestation?

    b.   Which fetus(es) is/are engaged?

    c.   Who is likely to deliver soonest? Why?

2. What is the primary reason for observing the bladder closely immediately after birth?

Student Name _____

CASE STUDIES

1. A nurse working in a prenatal clinic must teach a woman when to go to the hospital. The woman is having her third baby. Her first labor lasted 18 hours and her second labor lasted 6 hours. What should the nurse teach this woman? Give a rationale for each part of your teaching.

2. A woman is in labor with her first baby. Her cervix is 7 cm dilated, and the fetal station is +1. Formulate appropriate nursing interventions for the nursing diagnosis Pain related to labor process and exertion of labor.

APPLYING KNOWLEDGE

1. Use a model of a pelvis and fetal head to place the head in each of the following positions. Move the head through each mechanism of labor for each of the positions.

   a. ROA   d. LOA   f. LOP

   b. ROT   e. LOT   g. OA

   c. ROP

2. During your clinical experience, note how different fetal presentations or positions affect the woman's comfort during labor. Note if there is an apparent effect on the length of labor.

3. Palpate the uterine contractions of women in labor and classify them as mild, moderate, or firm intensity. Confirm your observations with an experienced intrapartum nurse.

4. Observe the labor of a woman having a vaginal birth after cesarean (VBAC) for the following factors related to her experience.
   a. number of previous cesarean and vaginal births
   b. reason for previous cesarean birth
   c. the woman's desire to have this baby vaginally
   d. maternal behaviors during labor
   e. support of her partner
   f. her apparent feelings after birth, whether it was VBAC or a repeat cesarean

5. Examine electronic fetal monitor strips to identify the following features:
   a. information that the monitor automatically prints on the strip (or the screen)
   b. interface with computer device, if any
   c. differences in appearance between those obtained with external devices and those from internal devices
   d. presence or absence of variability, rate accelerations, and deceleration patterns
   e. nursing and medical responses to abnormal patterns; fetal response to interventions
   f. outcome of birth, including Apgar scores of the infant

6. Locate the "precip tray" (which may have a different name) in your clinical facility. What are the contents of this tray?

REVIEW QUESTIONS

(136, 140) **1.** During labor, a fetal heart rate of 125–135 BPM should be interpreted as

    1. probably normal.
    2. possibly abnormal.
    3. probably abnormal.
    4. clearly abnormal.

(124, 126) **2.** When assessing the duration of labor contractions, the nurse should time from the

    1. beginning of one contraction to the end of the same contraction.
    2. end of one contraction to the beginning of the next.
    3. beginning of one contraction to the beginning of the next.
    4. peak of one contraction to the end of the contraction.

(145-146) **3.** During normal labor, contractions characteristically become

    1. more frequent and of shorter duration.
    2. more frequent and of longer duration.
    3. less frequent and of shorter duration.
    4. less frequent and of longer duration.

(141) **4.** When the fetus is in a cephalic presentation, the amniotic fluid is expected to be

    1. cloudy.   2. clear.
    3. green.   4. yellow.

(124) **5.** The thinning of the cervix during labor is called

    1. dilation.   2. effacement.
    3. station.   4. presentation.

(128-130) **6.** How should the nurse interpret the abbreviation ROP?

    1. The fetal sacrum is in the mother's right posterior pelvis.
    2. The fetal pelvis is in the mother's right occipital pelvis.
    3. The fetal occiput is in the mother's right posterior pelvis.
    4. The right fetal occiput is in the mother's posterior pelvis.

(145-146) **7.** The labor phase when the woman often feels anxious, restless, and seems to lose control is

    1. latent.   2. active.
    3. transition.   4. placental.

(150) **8.** Thirty minutes after birth, the nurse assesses the woman's uterine fundus. It is firm, above her umbilicus, and deviated to the right side. The appropriate nursing action is to

    1. massage the uterus.
    2. assist her to urinate.
    3. provide mild analgesia.
    4. restrict oral intake.

(128-130) **9.** Choose the abbreviation that describes the fetus in a breech presentation.

    1. LSA   2. OA
    3. ROA   4. LMT

(131) **10.** Which sign or symptom normally occurs shortly before labor begins?

    1. an urge to push or bear down
    2. increased clear vaginal discharge
    3. moderate amount of vaginal bleeding
    4. sudden weight gain of 3–5 pounds

Student Name _____

(131) **11.** Fetal descent during labor is measured in relation to the mother's

1. posterior perineum.
2. sacral promontory.
3. ischial spines.
4. uterine fundus.

(148) **12.** When the placenta is delivered with the fetal side presenting, the mechanism is called

1. Duncan.   2. Lamaze.
3. VBAC.   4. Schultz.

(145) **13.** During the latent phase of labor, the nurse should expect the woman's behavior to be

1. sleepy, except during contractions.
2. mildly anxious, coping with contractions.
3. quiet, concentrating on each contraction.
4. frustrated, losing control with contractions.

(141) **14.** A woman's membranes rupture during labor. The nurse notes that the fluid is yellowish and cloudy. The priority nursing response related to this assessment is to

1. remove wet underpads and replace them with dry ones.
2. perform a vaginal examination to assess labor progress.
3. reassure the woman that membrane rupture is expected.
4. assess the woman's temperature and the fetal heart rate.

(142) **15.** The nurse should learn to evaluate labor progress by methods other than vaginal examination, primarily because vaginal examination

1. worsens the mother's discomfort.
2. increases the risk for infection.
3. reduces fetal heart rate variability.
4. delays normal progression of labor.

(144, 146) **16.** Of those listed here, which is the priority nursing care during the second stage of labor?

1. Observe the woman's perineum.
2. Encourage pushing with contractions.
3. Evaluate labor coping skills.
4. Administer ordered analgesia.

(141, 154) **17.** Which maternal position should be avoided during labor?

1. sitting   2. walking
3. side-lying   4. supine

(144) **18.** The woman having a vaginal birth after cesarean (VBAC) should be observed during labor particularly for signs of

1. labor progression.
2. uterine rupture.
3. perineal pressure.
4. excessive anxiety.

(124) **19.** Which nursing assessment finding should be promptly reported to the physician or nurse-midwife?

1. clear amniotic fluid containing white flecks
2. fetal heart rate of 144 BPM with variability
3. vaginal discharge of mucus with dark blood
4. contractions that last longer than 90 seconds

(148) **20.** The priority nursing observation during the fourth stage is for

1. vaginal bleeding.
2. perineal bulging.
3. uterine infection.
4. parent-infant bonding.

(124) **21.** When assessing labor contractions, the nurse notes that the contracting uterus can be slightly indented with the fingertips when contractions are at their peak. Contraction intensity should be recorded as

1. mild.   2. moderate.
3. firm.   4. latent.

(133, 144) **22.** A woman phones the birth center and says, "I think my water broke, but I'm not having any contractions." The most appropriate nursing response is to tell her that

1. labor should begin within a few hours at most.
2. urine leakage is often confused with ruptured membranes.
3. she should come to the birth center for evaluation.
4. there is no concern unless the fluid is bloody.

(141) **23.** Amniotic fluid usually turns Nitrazine paper

1. yellow.   2. green.
3. dark blue.   4. purple.

(139-140) **24.** The nurse notes a pattern of variable decelerations on the electronic fetal monitor strip. The initial nursing response should be to

1. reassure the woman that the pattern is expected.
2. change the laboring woman's position.
3. increase the rate of the nonadditive IV fluid.
4. notify the physician of the abnormal pattern.

(149-150) **25.** The primary means to identify hemorrhage after vaginal birth is to

1. assess the vital signs frequently.
2. observe the uterine fundus and lochia.
3. keep an ice pack on the perineum.
4. have the woman urinate every 2 hours.

Student Name _____

● **CROSSWORD PUZZLE**

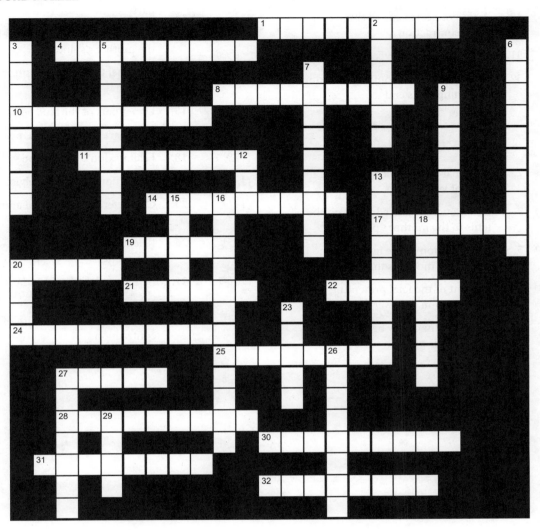

Across

(124, 126) **1.** Strength of labor contractions

(124, 126) **4.** Time interval from the beginning of one contraction until the beginning of the next

(132, 133) **8.** Pivoting of fetal head on the mother's symphysis pubis during labor

(124, 126) **10.** Period of increasing strength of a labor contraction

(132-133) **11.** Fetal rotation as the fetal head turns within the mother's pelvis

(127) **14.** Middle part of the true pelvis

(131, 133) **17.** Level of the fetal presenting part in relation to the ischial spines in the pelvis

(126) **19.** Part of the pelvis that is the upper flaring portion

(146, 148) **20.** Stage of labor from the baby's birth until delivery of the placenta

(127) **21.** Part of the true pelvis that is nearest the perineum

(141) **22.** Fetal substance that may normally be found in amniotic fluid

(124) **24.** Thinning of the cervix

(127) **25.** Fontanel that has four suture lines leading to it

(145) **27.** Stage of labor from its onset to complete cervical dilation

(132-133) **28.** Birth of the fetal shoulders and body

(124, 126) **30.** Period of decreasing strength of a labor contraction

(124) **31.** Opening of the cervix

(124) **32.** Length of a labor contraction from its beginning to its end

Down

(125) **2.** Maternal pushing occurs during this stage of labor

(128-129) **3.** Orientation of a fixed point on the fetus to the mother's pelvis

(132-133) **5.** Fetal rotation as the head turns to face one of the mother's thighs

(131, 133) **6.** Descent of the fetal presenting part to a zero station or lower

(141) **7.** Amniotic fluid may be cloudy if this condition is present

(131) **9.** Downward progress of fetal presenting part

(126-127) **12.** Orientation of the fetus in relation to the mother's spine

(127) **13.** Fontanel that has three suture lines leading to it

(126-127) **15.** Upper part of the true pelvis

(128) **16.** Fetal part that enters the pelvis first

(128) **18.** Fetal flexion or extension

(126) **20.** Lower portion of the pelvis

(141) **23.** Characteristic of normal amniotic fluid

(125) **26.** Relaxation period between two labor contractions

(131-133) **27.** Bending of the fetal head toward the chest

(124) **29.** Period of greatest strength of a labor contraction

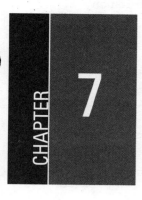

CHAPTER 7

Student Name _____

Nursing Management of Pain During Labor and Birth

Answer Key: Textbook page references are provided as a guide for answering these questions. A complete answer key was provided for your instructor.

LEARNING ACTIVITIES

1. Match the terms in the left column with their definitions on the right (a–e).

(162) _____ effleurage

(160) _____ endorphins

(162) _____ focal point

(158) _____ pain threshold

(158) _____ pain tolerance

a. least amount of stimulation that a person perceives as painful

b. maximum amount of pain one is willing to bear

c. stroking of the abdomen, thighs, or other body parts

d. intense concentration on an object

e. internal substances similar to morphine

(160) **2.** List four physical factors that cause pain during labor.

a. _____

b. _____

c. _____

d. _____

(160) **3.** How do each of these factors influence a woman's pain during labor?

a. Cervical readiness _____

_____

b. Pelvic size and shape _____

_____

c. Labor intensity _____

_____

    d.   Maternal fatigue _____

_____

    e.   Fetal presentation and position _____

_____

(158, 161) **4.** How does a woman's anxiety or fear relate to labor pain?

_____

_____

(158)   **5.** How can each aspect of prenatal classes help a woman in labor?

    a.   Education about expected changes _____

_____

    b.   Conditioning exercise _____

_____

(161)   **6.** List three reasons why it is useful for any laboring woman to know nonpharmacologic pain control methods.

    a. _____

    b. _____

    c. _____

(161-162) **7.** a. Explain why promoting a woman's relaxation during labor is essential to any type of pain management.

_____

_____

    b.   Describe at least four ways to help the laboring woman relax.

_____

_____

_____

_____

Student Name_____

(163, 164) **8.** What nursing care may help a woman cope with the following problems during labor?

a. Hyperventilation _____

_____

b. Urge to push before complete cervical dilation _____

_____

(164-165) **9.** Explain the differences between these anesthesia professionals.

a. Anesthesiologist _____

_____

b. Certified registered nurse-anesthetist (CRNA) _____

_____

(165) **10.** Explain why it is usually best to avoid opioid narcotic analgesics if birth is expected within 1 hour of administration.

_____

_____

_____

(165) **11.** What is the purpose of naloxone (Narcan)? What is an important nursing observation of the newborn related to use of this drug?

_____

_____

_____

12. For each type of regional anesthetic listed below, describe (a) how it is administered, (b) the location of its pain relief, (c) its major side effects, and (d) medical and nursing measures related to its use.

(167) **Local infiltration**

a. _____

_____

b. _____

_____

c.   _____

_____

d.   _____

_____

_____

(167-168)   **Pudendal block**

a.   _____

_____

b.   _____

_____

c.   _____

_____

d.   _____

_____

_____

(168-169)   **Epidural block**

a.   _____

_____

b.   _____

_____

c.   _____

_____

d.   _____

_____

_____

Student Name_____

(167) **Intrathecal analgesics**

a. _____

_____

b. _____

_____

c. _____

_____

d. _____

_____

_____

(169-170) **Subarachnoid block**

a. _____

_____

b. _____

_____

c. _____

_____

d. _____

_____

_____

(168) **13.** An anesthesiologist gives a test dose of the anesthetic agent when starting an epidural block to identify _____.

The expected reaction to the test dose is _____.

(167, 170) **14.** The woman who plans to have epidural anesthesia during labor and birth should be particularly questioned about allergy to _____.

Why? _____

(166-170) **15.** What is potentially the most life-threatening complication of general anesthesia for the mother? What is done to reduce the risk?

_____

_____

_____

THINKING CRITICALLY

1. Why do you think general anesthesia is almost never used for vaginal delivery in the United States or Canada?

2. A woman who is 2 hours postpartum after an uncomplicated birth wants to go to the bathroom to urinate. She had an epidural block for pain relief during labor and the medication and catheter for the block were removed immediately after birth. The infant has been nursing at intervals and the mother has eaten a light meal.

    a. Should you allow her to use the bathroom or have her use a bedpan? Explain the reason for your choice.

    b. If you allow her to walk to the bathroom, describe what you should do to ensure her safety.

CASE STUDIES

1. a. Jill Sims is a primigravida in labor at 4 cm cervical dilation. She is using breathing techniques she learned in prepared childbirth classes. Jill is breathing rapidly throughout each contraction. She complains of stiff fingers and numbness around her mouth. What is the probable cause of Jill's symptoms? What is an appropriate nursing measure to help correct her problem?
    b. Jill is now 5–6 cm dilated and requests an epidural block. Is this an appropriate time during labor to give an epidural block? If so, what nursing observations are most important before and after the block is begun?
    c. What nursing measures are appropriate during second-stage labor?

2. You are working with a laboring woman and note that she is holding her body stiffly and gripping the bed rails tightly during each contraction. What nursing interventions are appropriate in each of the following areas? (This activity can be used to demonstrate the techniques for a clinical postconference. If so, suggest other techniques.)
    a. Relaxation techniques
    b. Adjusting the environment
    c. Assisting her with breathing techniques

Student Name _____

APPLYING KNOWLEDGE

1. When you are in the hospital, look at trays used to administer various anes[...] the following components in the trays.
   a. pudendal block tray: trumpet
   b. epidural block tray: Touhy or other needle used to insert into the epidu[...] space, epidural catheter
   c. subarachnoid (spinal) block tray: spinal needle (note any size difference from the epidural needle)

2. Identify professionals in your hospital who administer obstetrical anesthesia. Are they limited to administration of specific types of anesthesia? Is one present 24 hours a day? Do obstetricians give epidural blocks?

3. Look at the contents of emergency carts for women and newborns. Who usually handles emergency care of newborns who are in distress? Do they hold certification from the American Heart Association and American Academy of Pediatrics in neonatal resuscitation (NRP)? Which professionals are present at uncomplicated births or cesarean births to care for the infant?

4. What is the most common anesthesia for vaginal birth in your hospital? For cesarean birth?

5. Observe a childbirth education class.

6. Observe a laboring woman using childbirth preparation techniques. Who is her support person? How is the support person helping her use these techniques? How can you help her?

REVIEW QUESTIONS

(160) 1. According to the gate control theory, which technique should be most helpful in interrupting transmission of labor pain to the brain?
   1. rapid, shallow breathing
   2. application of heat
   3. focusing on a point in the room
   4. deep cleansing breaths

(161, 164) 2. Choose the best method during the admission process to help relieve general anxiety for a woman having her first baby who has not attended prepared childbirth classes.
   1. Assure her that she will be given pain medication any time she needs it.
   2. Determine her reasons for not attending the classes offered in the hospital.
   3. Have her take deep breaths to relax all muscles before doing any admission assessments.
   4. Give simple explanations about her environment and what to expect during labor.

(165) **3.** Butorphanol differs from meperidine in that butorphanol

1. should not be used if a woman is dependent on heroin.
2. causes greater respiratory depression in the newborn.
3. better reduces the pain of late labor.
4. cannot be reversed with naloxone.

(165, 167) **4.** The newborn of a woman who receives narcotic analgesics during labor should be observed primarily for

1. convulsions.
2. slow respirations.
3. excess activity.
4. constipation.

(167-169) **5.** A woman (gravida 2, para 1) plans an epidural block for labor and birth. Which factor in her history is most significant in terms of her planned anesthetic?

1. mild hypertension during first pregnancy
2. light meal 4 hours before labor began
3. forceps delivery during first birth
4. adverse reaction to dental anesthetic

(166, 168) **6.** An advantage of an epidural block is that it

1. reduces pain for both labor and birth.
2. has no fetal or maternal risks.
3. supports normal blood pressure.
4. enhances the woman's urge to push.

(166, 167) **7.** Immediately after birth, nursing care for the woman who had subarachnoid block anesthesia for a repeat cesarean birth should include

1. ambulating within 2 hours of birth.
2. keeping her back curved outward.
3. assessing for return of sensation.
4. keeping her flat in bed for 8 hours.

(170) **8.** A blood patch may be done to relieve

1. low blood pressure.
2. respiratory depression.
3. postspinal headache.
4. prolonged numbness.

(174) **9.** The nurse should observe the woman who received epidural opioid narcotics for

1. late respiratory depression.
2. nausea and vomiting.
3. unstable blood pressure.
4. persistent headache.

(166) **10.** During general anesthesia, cricoid pressure is done to

1. reduce stomach acid secretion.
2. avoid aspiration of gastric contents.
3. prevent excessive blood loss.
4. limit musculoskeletal injuries.

(161-164) **11.** A woman asks if she should take prepared childbirth classes. The best response of the nurse is to tell her that classes will

1. allow her to avoid pain medications during labor.
2. be required if her partner wants to be with her.
3. provide methods to help her cope with labor.
4. reduce the likelihood that complications will occur.

Student Name _____

(162) 12. The prepared childbirth technique that is most likely to relieve back pain during labor is

1. effleurage.
2. sacral pressure.
3. thermal stimulation.
4. patterned breathing.

(163-164) 13. A woman is using prepared childbirth breathing techniques and complains of dizziness and tingling. The nurse should

1. have her breathe more rapidly with contractions.
2. ask her if she feels an urge to push or bear down.
3. tell her to exhale slowly into her cupped hands.
4. reassure her that these sensations are normal.

(172) 14. Immediately after an epidural block is begun, the woman may be positioned

1. flat on her back, with no pillow.
2. sitting upright with her legs over the side of the bed.
3. with a small roll under her right hip.
4. in a modified Trendelenburg position.

(166, 171) 15. Two hours after a vaginal birth with an epidural anesthesia, the nurse determines that the woman's bladder is full. The most appropriate initial nursing action is to

1. help her walk to the bathroom if movement and sensation have returned.
2. ask her how full her bladder feels before allowing her to walk to the bathroom.
3. insert an indwelling (Foley) catheter until the woman is at least 8 hours postpartum.
4. take no action unless the woman says her full bladder makes her uncomfortable.

(166, 174) 16. The most effective way to identify adequate maternal oxygenation after general anesthesia for cesarean birth is to

1. take the blood pressure regularly.
2. observe for cyanosis or restlessness.
3. maintain a side-lying position.
4. observe pulse-oximeter readings.

Student Name _____

CHAPTER 8

Nursing Care of Women with Complications During Labor and Birth

Answer Key: Textbook page references are provided as a guide for answering these questions. A complete answer key was provided for your instructor.

LEARNING ACTIVITIES

1. Match the terms in the left column with their definitions on the right (a–h).

(176)	_____ amniotomy	a. infection of the amniotic sac
(183)	_____ cephalopelvic disproportion	b. excessive amniotic fluid
		c. substance that swells within the cervix, dilating it slightly
(183)	_____ chignon	d. circular swelling on the neonate's head caused by vacuum extractor
(196)	_____ chorioamnionitis	e. large body size
(188)	_____ dystocia	f. artificial rupture of the amniotic sac
(177)	_____ hydramnios	g. inability of the fetus to fit through the pelvis
		h. difficult labor
(178)	_____ laminaria	
(192)	_____ macrosomia	

(176-177) **2.** Describe three potential complications of amniotomy and the nursing assessments that should be reported for each.

a. _____

_____

_____

b. _____

_____

_____

c. _____

_____

_____

(177)   **3.**   Distinguish between labor *induction* and labor *augmentation.*

_____

_____

_____

4.   Identify each drug or class of drugs from the following descriptions of their main purpose. Give examples of specific drugs for c and d.

(178)   a.   Soften the cervix _____

_____

(179)   b.   Stimulate labor contractions _____

_____

(197)   c.   Inhibit uterine contractions _____

_____

(197-198)   d.   Speed fetal lung maturation _____

_____

(181-182) **5.**   Describe three nursing measures to promote comfort in a woman who has an episiotomy or perineal laceration.

a. _____

b. _____

c. _____

(184-185) **6.**   Two separate incisions are done in cesarean delivery. What are they? Which of the two is more important and why?

_____

_____

_____

Student Name_____

(185, 187) **7.** What nursing observations are appropriate after cesarean birth in each of the following areas and why?

a. Vital signs and other monitor output (pulse oximeter, etc.) _____

_____

b. IV fluid _____

_____

c. Uterine fundus _____

_____

d. Dressing _____

_____

e. Lochia _____

_____

f. Indwelling catheter _____

_____

(188, 190) **8.** Compare *hypotonic* labor to *hypertonic* labor for the following characteristics. Note which one is most common.

Characteristic	Hypotonic Labor	Hypertonic Labor
Contractions		
Time of occurrence during labor		
Medical management		
Nursing care		

9. Describe how each of the following factors can contribute to abnormal labor and list nursing measures appropriate for each.

(190-192)   a. Ineffective pushing efforts _____

_____

_____

_____

_____

(193)   b. Occiput posterior fetal position _____

_____

_____

_____

_____

(195)   10. State four ways that excessive psychological stress can contribute to a difficult labor.

_____

_____

_____

_____

(195)   11. Describe four possible adverse effects of prolonged labor on either the mother or the fetus.

a. _____

b. _____

c. _____

d. _____

(195-196) 12. Describe possible adverse effects of precipitous labor on the mother and fetus.

a. _____

b. _____

c. _____

Student Name_____

(196)   **13.** What is the difference between PROM and PPROM?

_____

_____

_____

_____

(196, 198) **14.** What is the role of each of the following measures in the care of the woman with threatened or actual preterm labor?

a.   Transvaginal ultrasound _____

_____

b.   Activity restrictions _____

_____

c.   Fetal fibronectin _____

_____

(197)   **15.** Describe at least five symptoms of preterm labor that should be taught to every pregnant woman.

_____

_____

_____

_____

_____

_____

(198)   **16.** Describe nursing care of the fetus or neonate related to these problems of prolonged pregnancy.

a.   Placental blood supply _____

_____

b.   Passage of meconium in utero _____

_____

c.   Consumption of glucose reserves prior to birth _____

_____

(198-199) **17.** Describe four situations in which the nurse must be especially watchful for a prolapsed umbilical cord.

a.   _____

b.   _____

c.   _____

d.   _____

(199)   **18.** Describe three variations of uterine rupture.

a.   _____

_____

b.   _____

_____

c.   _____

_____

THINKING CRITICALLY

1.   In addition to assessing the progress of labor, what other nursing assessments are important for the woman who has a precipitous labor? How can positioning the woman on her side improve the fetus's oxygen supply?

CASE STUDIES

1.   Cara Miller is a 24-year-old gravida 2, para 1, who is in early labor with her first baby. Her cervix is 3 cm dilated and 75% effaced; fetal station is 0. Contractions are every 4 minutes, 30–35 seconds in duration, and of moderate intensity. The nurse-midwife performs an amniotomy. A small amount of light-green fluid drains on the underpad.
  a.   Use your birth facility's standard form to chart this information about Cara's labor.
  b.   Is there significance to the color of the amniotic fluid? If so, what is the significance?
  c.   What nursing interventions are appropriate specific to the situation above? What other person or persons, if any, in your facility should be notified of these findings?
  d.   Describe observations that would suggest that the amniotomy caused complications of any kind.

Student Name_____

2. Baby boy Briggs was born in a forceps-assisted birth. What observations should the nurse make in each area listed below? What observations would be significant in terms of complications?
   a. skin
   b. shape of head
   c. appearance when crying

3. Write a simple explanation to parents about the appearance of the infant's head if the birth was assisted with a vacuum extractor.

APPLYING KNOWLEDGE

1. Observe newborns who were in abnormal presentations or positions before birth. Identify characteristics caused by the abnormal presentation or position.

2. What nursing interventions do nurses in your clinical setting use when a mother is having complicated labor? How did you contribute to a mother's physical or psychological comfort during labor? What was the reason for the woman's abnormal labor?

3. What drugs to stop preterm labor are prescribed in your clinical setting? Read the policies and procedures related to administration of the drugs. If possible, assist in the care of a woman who is receiving the drugs. What concerns do the woman and her family express?

4. Make a list of activities appropriate for a woman on activity restriction for preterm labor, both in the hospital and at home.

5. Observe a woman who has a cesarean birth after labor, focusing on her feelings about the surgical birth. Compare your observations with those of classmates who have cared for other women who had scheduled cesarean births.

REVIEW QUESTIONS

(177) 1. After amniotomy, which of the following observations should be reported immediately?

1. clear fluid draining on the underpad
2. maternal temperature of 37.2°C (99.0°F)
3. fetal heart rate of 95 BPM
4. moderate contractions every 3 minutes

(188, 190) 2. Which is the most appropriate nursing care for the woman having hypertonic labor?

1. Encourage walking in the hallway to improve contractions and enhance labor.
2. Promote rest and provide general comfort measures.
3. Reassure her that this problem will go away when active labor begins.
4. Omit oral fluids and increase the rate of intravenous fluid.

(188, 190) **3.** A woman, gravida 4, para 3, has been 5 cm dilated for 2 hours. Her contractions are every 7 minutes, 30 seconds duration, and mild. The FHR is 135–145/minute. She is relatively comfortable. This woman is most likely experiencing

1. hypotonic labor dysfunction.
2. hypertonic labor dysfunction.
3. occiput posterior fetal position.
4. fetal shoulder dystocia.

(195-196) **4.** The most desirable position for a woman having a precipitous labor is

1. side-lying.
2. semi-Fowler's.
3. Trendelenburg.
4. hands and knees.

(193) **5.** After a vaginal birth complicated by shoulder dystocia, the nurse should particularly assess the newborn for

1. molding of the head.
2. flexed positioning.
3. clavicle deformity.
4. abnormal temperature.

(197-198) **6.** A woman has ruptured membranes at 35 weeks gestation. Which nursing observation should be promptly reported?

1. FHR: accelerations present; average rate of 135–145 BPM
2. clear, nonirritating vaginal discharge
3. occasional spontaneous fetal movement
4. slight crackles heard with lung assessment

(193) **7.** Which is the most typical labor characteristic when the fetus is in an occiput posterior position?

1. labor length under 3 hours
2. persistent back discomfort
3. rapid fetal descent
4. mild contraction strength

(197) **8.** A woman who is at 32 weeks gestation telephones the nurse in a labor unit and says that her baby seems to be "pushing down" much of the time and that she has a constant backache. Choose the most appropriate nursing response.

1. Ask her to have someone bring her to the labor unit for further assessment.
2. Reassure her that pressure and backache are common during late pregnancy.
3. Tell her she should rest with her feet elevated several times each day.
4. Encourage her to promote bladder emptying by increasing her fluid intake.

(180) **9.** External version is most likely to be done in which of these situations?

1. early labor with frank breech presentation
2. breech presentation with placenta previa
3. twins in cephalic and breech presentations
4. breech presentation at 38 weeks gestation

(198-199) **10.** The first nursing action if a visibly prolapsed umbilical cord occurs is to

1. call the physician or nurse-midwife.
2. palpate the cord for a pulse.
3. apply the internal fetal monitor.
4. relieve pressure on the cord.

177) **11.** What is the priority nursing action following amniotomy?

1. Turn the woman to her side.
2. Check the fetal heart rate.
3. Assess the color of the fluid.
4. Change the underpad.

Student Name_____

(181-182) **12.** The nursing intervention most likely to make the woman with a perineal laceration more comfortable during the first 2 hours after birth is

1. warm-water soaks.
2. a small dressing.
3. an ice pack.
4. antibacterial ointment.

(182-183) **13.** The parents of a newborn delivered with low forceps ask about small bruises on each side of the baby's head. The nurse should tell the parents that the bruises

1. will be reported to the physician.
2. usually disappear in a few days.
3. may indicate brain damage.
4. occur in all deliveries.

(185) **14.** The most important nursing care during the recovery period after cesarean birth is to

1. provide analgesia.
2. assess the fundus.
3. position for comfort.
4. encourage urination.

(199-200) **15.** When caring for a woman following a car accident at 36 weeks of pregnancy, what is the priority fetal assessment?

1. undetected trauma
2. poor oxygenation
3. intrauterine infection
4. precipitous birth

(199-200) **16.** The nurse must particularly observe for signs and symptoms of uterine rupture if the laboring woman has

1. a hypotonic labor pattern.
2. a prior cesarean birth.
3. prematurely ruptured membranes.
4. estimated fetal weight of 3500 g.

(198) **17.** An infant's amniotic fluid was meconium-stained. During the admission assessment, the nurse notes that the infant is crying vigorously. Her skin is peeling and she has a long, thin appearance. These facts suggest that this infant is probably

1. preterm.
2. postterm.
3. in respiratory distress.
4. large for her gestation.

(178) **18.** A woman has prostaglandin gel applied to her cervix the day before she is scheduled for induction of labor at 40 weeks. Which is the most appropriate teaching before she returns home?

1. Do not eat or drink anything until you return for labor induction.
2. Your bag of waters will probably rupture before you return tomorrow.
3. Return to the birth center if you begin having regular contractions.
4. Stay in bed, lying on your left side, until you return for labor induction.

(183-184) **19.** An infant is born by elective (planned) cesarean birth because of a breech presentation. The infant weighs 3206 g (7 pounds, 1 ounce). The nursery nurse should particularly observe this infant for

1. low blood sugar.
2. respiratory difficulty.
3. birth injury.
4. generalized infection.

CHAPTER 9

The Family After Birth

Answer Key: Textbook page references are provided as a guide for answering these questions. A complete answer key was provided for your instructor.

LEARNING ACTIVITIES

(205) **1.** Describe the following expected assessments for the uterine fundus immediately after birth.

   a. Location _____

   _____

   b. Consistency _____

(205, 206) **2.** Describe the initial nursing action if the fundus is boggy (soft) and bleeding is excessive during the postpartum period. How does this action control uterine bleeding?

   _____

   _____

(206) **3.** List two drugs that may be ordered to correct uterine atony and the acceptable routes of administration.

   a. _____

   b. _____

(205-206) **4.** List and describe the three stages of lochia, including approximate time periods for each.

   a. _____

   _____

   b. _____

   _____

   c. _____

   _____

(208)   **5.**   When should perineal care be done?

a.   _____

b.   _____

(208)   **6.**   What should the nurse teach a postpartum woman about doing perineal care and about applying and removing her perineal pad? Why is it important to do these procedures in this way?

_____

_____

(208)   **7.**   a.   The new mother can expect her menstrual periods to resume in

_____ weeks if she is not breastfeeding.

b.   In the breastfeeding mother, return of ovulation and menstruation are

_____ .

(209)   **8.**   Average blood loss at birth is about _____ for vaginal birth and

_____ for cesarean birth.

(209)   **9.**   Describe two nursing actions that may make a woman who is chilled and shaking after birth more comfortable.

a.   _____

b.   _____

(210)   **10.**   Describe two possible signs of a full bladder in the immediate postpartum period.

a.   Height of uterus _____

b.   Location of uterus _____

(210)   **11.**   Describe five nursing actions to help a new mother to empty her bladder after birth.

a.   _____

b.   _____

c.   _____

d.   _____

e.   _____

Student Name_____

(210) **12.** List three nursing measures to prevent or correct constipation after birth.

a. _____

b. _____

c. _____

(211) **13.** Describe each of the following factors about postbirth use of $Rh_o(D)$ immune globulin (RhoGAM).

a. Mother's Rh factor _____

b. Infant's Rh factor _____

c. Recommended time of administration after birth_____

d. Site and route of administration _____

(211-213) **14.** Explain each of the following factors about postpartum rubella immunization.

a. Why it is given to the nonimmune woman at this time? _____

_____

b. Precautions _____

_____

c. Safety during breastfeeding _____

_____

(211-213) **15.** What assessments should the nurse make in each of these areas when caring for the woman who has had a cesarean birth?

a. Uterine fundus _____

_____

b. Lochia _____

_____

c. Dressing _____

_____

d. Urinary output _____

_____

(214)   **16.** Name and describe Rubin's three postpartum psychological phases.

    a.   _____

        _____

    b.   _____

        _____

    c.   _____

        _____

(214)   **17.** What are the appropriate nursing interventions for postpartum blues?

        _____

        _____

(215-216) **18.** Describe nursing interventions that may be appropriate for grieving families in the maternity setting.

        _____

        _____

        _____

        _____

(218)   **19.** Describe newborn behaviors during each stage of transition and the approximate duration of each stage.

    a.   First stage _____

        _____

    b.   Second stage _____

        _____

    c.   Third stage _____

        _____

(218)   **20.** Why is prevention of neonatal hypothermia particularly important?

        _____

        _____

        _____

Student Name_____

●

(221)   **21.**   The nurse should normally be able to identify how many arteries are in the newborn's

umbilical cord? _____ How many veins? _____ What word can be

used to help remember these numbers? _____

(221-222) **22.** a.   What is the minimum normal blood glucose on screening tests for a newborn (include

units of measure)? _____

b.   List signs of hypoglycemia in a newborn.

_____

_____

_____

(222)   **23.**   List seven common laboratory screening tests for newborns. Identify the one that is manda-
tory in all states.

●

a.   _____

b.   _____

c.   _____

d.   _____

e.   _____

f.   _____

g.   _____

(222-223) **24.**   List three types of parent-infant contact that enhance attachment. Which of these is most
important?

a.   _____

b.   _____

c.   _____

(226)   **25.** a.   Describe colostrum.

●

_____

_____

b.   Explain the neonatal benefits of colostrum. _____

_____

(230)   **26.**   Describe methods to prevent and relieve breast engorgement.

_____

_____

_____

(232)   **27.**   Describe the following nutritional needs of the breastfeeding mother.

a.   Calories _____

b.   Foods _____

c.   Fluids _____

d.   Supplements_____

(232)   **28.**   What should the nurse teach the breastfeeding mother in each of the following areas?

a.   Foods that the infant may not tolerate_____

_____

b.   Medications _____

_____

(232-233) **29.**   List four types of infant formula. Give an example of the three main types.

a.   _____

b.   _____

c.   _____

d.   _____

(233)   **30.**   Describe the three common forms for infant formulas.

_____

_____

_____

Student Name_____

(233-234) **31.** Describe teaching in each of the following areas for bottle-feeding parents.

     a.   Propping the bottle _____

     b.   Size of nipple holes _____

     c.   Warming and microwaving _____

         _____

     d.   Burping _____

     e.   Positioning baby after feeding _____

         _____

     f.   Leftover formula _____

(234) **32.** Describe appropriate nursing teaching in the following areas for postpartum discharge.

     a.   Hygiene _____

         _____

     b.   Sexual intercourse _____

         _____

     c.   Diet _____

         _____

(234-235) **33.** List nine danger signals that a postpartum woman should promptly report to her physician or nurse-midwife.

     a.   _____

     b.   _____

     c.   _____

     d.   _____

     e.   _____

     f.   _____

     g.   _____

     h.   _____

     i.   _____

(235) **34.** Describe the following factors about automobile safety.

a. Ideal position for infant _____

_____

b. When a forward-facing seat can be used _____

c. Securing infant in seat and seat to vehicle _____

_____

d. Air bag safety _____

_____

THINKING CRITICALLY

1. After a cesarean birth, what are some nursing interventions to help a mother manage pain while remaining alert enough to nurse her baby? Why is this mother likely to need additional nutrition teaching? What if her cesarean was done for placenta previa complicated by hemorrhage?

CASE STUDY

1. a. Cynthia Chung, 26 years old, expects her first baby in about 12 weeks. She says that she is having a difficult time deciding whether to breastfeed or bottle feed the baby. What information should you provide Cynthia to help her make this decision? What information would be available to use at your clinical facility?

   b. Cynthia decides to breastfeed her baby. On the fifth day after birth, she phones the unit to say that she has breast engorgement and her nipples are sore. Her left nipple has a small crack. What can the nurse teach Cynthia to help her cope with these problems?

   c. What should the nurse teach Cynthia about care of the baby's umbilical stump? What signs of problems should she report?

APPLYING KNOWLEDGE

1. What analgesics do postpartum women in your hospital receive for pain? Do nurses use any nonpharmacologic techniques to make the women more comfortable?

2. Observe families during the postpartum period. What interactions do you see between mother, father, and newborn? Identify practices in your clinical setting that enhance or inhibit parent-infant attachment.

3. Assist the staff nurse to help new mothers learn to breastfeed. If you have successfully breastfed a baby yourself, share appropriate helpful hints with new mothers and classmates.

(211)   7.   The nurse gives a postpartum woman a rubella immunization. Which is the most important patient teaching related to this immunization?

1. Neomycin can be used for rash or elevated temperature.
2. Use a reliable birth control method for 3 months.
3. Immunization now gives the baby immunity through breast milk.
4. Increased urination is a common side effect of the immunization.

(208)   8.   What should the mother be taught about perineal cleansing?

1. Do perineal cleansing only after bowel movements.
2. Cleanse from back to front with soft wipes.
3. Direct the flow of fluid from the front to the back.
4. Do not use disposable wipes on the perineal area.

(226)   9.   Colostrum's greatest benefit to the infant is prevention of

1. constipation.
2. weight loss.
3. hemorrhage.
4. infection.

(225)   10.   The let-down reflex is stimulated by

1. massage of the uterus.
2. suckling of the baby.
3. increased fluid intake.
4. breast engorgement.

(230)   11.   What should the nursing mother be taught about breast care?

1. Clean the breasts with plain water when washing.
2. Give one formula feeding daily to limit engorgement.
3. Do not wear a bra the first few days after birth.
4. Begin with the same breast at each feeding.

(233)   12.   Choose the best position for the newborn after feeding.

1. in an infant seat
2. on the abdomen
3. with upper body elevated
4. side-lying with head down

(205)   13.   At her 2-week postpartum check-up, the woman's uterus should be

1. two fingerwidths above the umbilicus.
2. two fingerwidths below the umbilicus.
3. just above the symphysis pubis.
4. no longer palpable through the abdomen.

(209)   14.   Diuresis in the early postpartum period indicates

1. urinary tract infection.
2. retention of body fluids.
3. excretion of excess fluid.
4. edema near the urinary meatus.

(207, 234)   15.   The earliest time when sexual intercourse can usually be resumed after birth is

1. at 2 weeks postpartum.
2. when the episiotomy heals.
3. when lochia alba is present.
4. after the 6-week check.

(219)   16.   The most appropriate way to identify mother and infant when reuniting them is to

1. check the identification band numbers of each.
2. ask the mother to clearly state her name.
3. examine the mother's fingerprint and infant's footprints.
4. verify that the names on the crib card and band are identical.

Student Name _____

(208) 17. Which is the best nursing measure to increase the woman's perineal comfort during the first hour after vaginal birth with a midline episiotomy?

　　1. Help her take a warm sitz bath.
　　2. Give her an oral analgesic drug.
　　3. Apply topical anesthetic ointment.
　　4. Place an ice pack on the area.

(230) 18. A mother phones the postpartum unit 4 days after birth. She says her baby cannot suck well on her nipples because her breasts are full and engorged. What should the nurse recommend?

　　1. Apply ice packs just before allowing the infant to nurse.
　　2. Feed formula for the next two feedings to reduce pain and congestion.
　　3. Massage the breasts and express a small amount of milk before nursing.
　　4. Reduce daily liquid intake to 1 quart for a few days.

(233-234) 19. The nurse notes that a new mother has several bottles of partly consumed formula on her overbed table. Choose the most appropriate nursing action.

　　1. Recommend that she prepare bottles that contain only what the baby is likely to drink.
　　2. Inform her that the bottles cannot be used because they have not been refrigerated.
　　3. Tell her she may combine the leftover formula for the baby's next feeding.
　　4. Check the room for other partially used bottles, then throw all of them in the trash.

(206-207) 20. Which lochia characteristic should the nurse teach the woman to report?

　　1. change from red to pink-brown to white
　　2. cessation of flow by 4 weeks postpartum
　　3. return of red flow at 12 days postpartum
　　4. presence of a menstrual-like odor

CROSSWORD PUZZLE

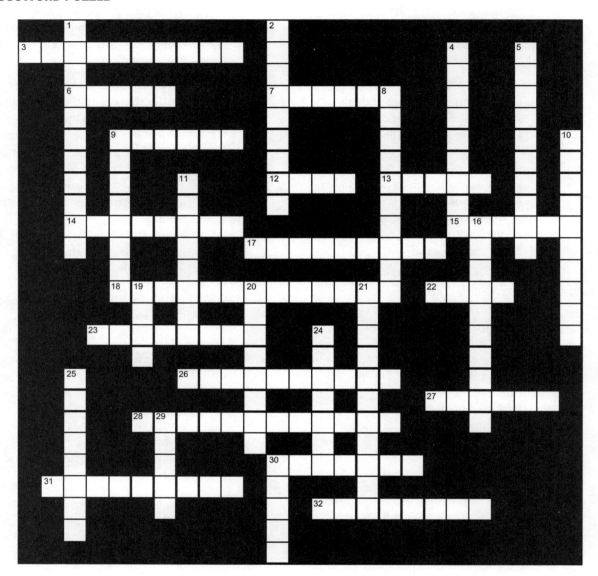

Across

(218) **3.** Type of heat loss caused when infant is placed on cool surface for assessment

(208) **6.** Acronym used for assessment of episiotomy or other incision

(205-206) **7.** Vaginal drainage after birth; has three stages

(206) **9.** Lochia that has a pink color

(219) **12.** Abbreviation for intrauterine growth restriction

(205-206) **13.** Bloody postpartum lochia

(213) **14.** Drug used to reverse respiratory depression caused by epidural narcotics

(226) **15.** Human milk having a bluish color

(218) **17.** Type of heat loss caused by locating infant's crib near a cold wall

(226) **18.** Breast milk enhancers used by some cultures

(235) **22.** Direction the infant should face in his or her car seat

(216) **23.** Mood instability

Student Name_____

(204) **26.** Return of the uterus to its normal state after birth

(205) **27.** Top of the uterus that contracts to control bleeding after birth

(226) **28.** Milk secreted after colostrum

(222) **30.** Strong emotional tie that develops soon after birth

(210) **31.** Separation of the longitudinal abdominal muscles (rectus muscles)

(226) **32.** Breast milk with higher fat content to satisfy infant's hunger

Down

(214) **1.** Father's intense interest in his new baby

(225) **2.** Anterior pituitary hormone that stimulates breasts to produce milk

(226) **4.** First breast secretion; high in antibodies

(203) **5.** First 6 weeks after birth

(205) **8.** Intermittent uterine contractions after birth, similar to menstrual cramps

(228) **9.** Giving or taking nourishment at the breast

(218) **10.** Type of heat loss caused by air-conditioning vent blowing air on infant

(227) **11.** Good infant hold for breastfeeding woman who had a cesarean birth

(223) **16.** Long-term affectional tie between the infant and parent

(206) **19.** Lochia that is mostly mucus

(225) **20.** Posterior pituitary hormone that causes let-down reflex and uterine contractions

(218) **21.** Type of heat loss caused when parent bathes infant slowly

(225) **24.** Reflex that ejects milk from alveoli to the ductal system of nipple

(226) **25.** Watery, thirst-quenching breast milk

(207) **29.** Vaginal folds

(214) **30.** Transient feelings of joy and emotional letdown after birth

CHAPTER 10

Student Name _____

Nursing Care of Women with Complications Following Birth

Answer Key: Textbook page references are provided as a guide for answering these questions. A complete answer key was provided for your instructor.

LEARNING ACTIVITIES

1. Match the terms in the left column with their definitions on the right (a–m).

(248)	_____ "baby blues"	a. infection of the uterine lining
(249)	_____ bipolar disorder	b. infection of the breast
(243)	_____ curettage	c. lodging of a blood clot in a blood vessel of the lung
(248)	_____ postpartum depression	d. calf pain when the foot is dorsiflexed
(244)	_____ endometritis	e. inadequate amount of blood to maintain normal circulation
(241)	_____ hematoma	f. mood disorder characterized by impairment of reality
(243)	_____ Homan's sign	g. mood disorder characterized by episodes of mania alternating with depression
(238)	_____ hypovolemic shock	h. hyperactive, excitable, euphoric behavior
(249)	_____ mania	i. delayed return of the uterus to its nonpregnant state
(246)	_____ mastitis	j. collection of blood within tissues
(248)	_____ psychosis	k. scraping or vacuuming the inner surface of the uterus
(243)	_____ pulmonary embolism	l. postpartum emotional state characterized by feelings of being let down, but generally satisfied with life
(247)	_____ subinvolution	m. nonpsychosis characterized by loss of enjoyment, lack of interest, feelings of inadequacy after birth

(237) 2. Postpartum hemorrhage is blood loss that exceeds _____ ml after vaginal birth or _____ ml after cesarean birth.

(237)   **3.**   Early postpartum hemorrhage occurs within _____ hours of birth; late postpartum

hemorrhage occurs later than _____ hours after birth until _____ weeks after birth.

(238)   **4.**   Describe the following five changes that occur in hypovolemic shock and indicate the change
or changes that usually occur early.

    a.   Heart rate _____

        _____

    b.   Respiratory rate _____

        _____

    c.   Blood pressure _____

        _____

    d.   Skin and mucous membranes _____

        _____

    e.   Mental state _____

        _____

(240)   **5.**   Why does a poorly contracted uterus lead to hemorrhage?

    _____

    _____

(241)   **6.**   What is the connection between the infant suckling at the breast and control of postpartum
bleeding?

    _____

    _____

(240-241)   **7.**   Describe typical differences in bleeding and uterine fundus characteristics between hemorrhage caused by uterine atony and that caused by a birth canal laceration.

    a.   Bleeding

        Uterine atony _____

        _____

        Laceration _____

        _____

Student Name_____

⬤

        b.   Uterine fundus

            Uterine atony _____

            _____

            _____

            Laceration _____

            _____

            _____

(241, 242) **8.**   Describe the following typical manifestations of a birth canal hematoma.

        a.   Visual appearance _____

            _____

        b.   Character of pain or pressure_____

            _____

            _____

⬤

        c.   Signs of blood loss _____

            _____

(243)   **9.**   How does manual removal of the placenta differ from the usual method of separation?

        _____

        _____

        _____

(243-244) **10.**   Distinguish between the characteristics of a superficial vein thrombosis (SVT) and a deep vein thrombosis (DVT).

        a.   Superficial vein thrombosis _____

            _____

        b.   Deep vein thrombosis _____

            _____

⬤ *(243-244)* **11.**   The greatest risk of deep vein thrombosis is that it may result in_____

        _____ .

(244) **12.** Postpartum infection is generally characterized by a temperature of _____

after the first _____ hours after birth, occurring on at least _____ days during

the first _____ days after birth.

(245) **13.** List the localized signs and symptoms of an infection such as a wound infection.

_____

_____

(244-246) **14.** Why are postpartum infections in the reproductive tract likely to spread?

_____

_____

(244) **15.** Why may the white blood cell (leukocyte) count be unreliable as the only assessment to diagnose infection after birth? _____

_____

(245-246) **16.** What nutritional information is important when teaching the woman who has—or is at an increased risk of having—a postpartum infection? Would this teaching be appropriate for other people with an infection?

_____

_____

_____

(245) **17.** Distinguish between *cystitis* and *pyelonephritis* in terms of the following characteristics. Which is the most serious?

a. Fever _____

_____

b. Discomfort _____

_____

_____

c. Other characteristics _____

_____

_____

Student Name_____

(245) **18.** Describe the following nursing measures to promote recovery from urinary tract infection and prevent future ones.

    a.   Fluid intake _____

        _____

    b.   Beneficial foods _____

        _____

(246) **19.** Which two factors increase the likelihood that mastitis will develop?

    a.   _____

    b.   _____

(246-247) **20.** What is the role of heat application in the care of a woman with mastitis?

    a.   _____

    b.   _____

    c.   _____

(247) **21.** Describe three characteristics of subinvolution of the uterus.

    a.   _____

        _____

    b.   _____

        _____

    c.   _____

        _____

(248) **22.** Describe the basic difference between postpartum "blues" and postpartum depression.

    a.   Postpartum "blues" _____

        _____

    b.   Postpartum depression _____

        _____

        _____

THINKING CRITICALLY

1. How can the nurse's teaching about breastfeeding reduce the likelihood that a woman will develop mastitis?

2. A woman is having her 6-week examination after a normal vaginal birth at the office where you work. She has a "flat" appearance to her face and seems uninterested in what you say to her, although she cooperates with each request related to her examination and cares for her baby when he cries. What possibilities for her behavior should you consider? How should you respond to her?

CASE STUDY

1. Carmen Esparza is transferred to the mother-baby unit after a cesarean delivery 2 hours ago following a long labor. Her healthy daughter weighs 4540 g (10 pounds). Carmen's blood loss during surgery was 1200 ml. Her vital signs on admission to the unit are: T 99, P 86, R 20, BP 118/80. Her fundus is firm, midline, and lochia is scant in amount. The dressing over her incision is clean and dry. The indwelling catheter bag contained 550 ml of light-yellow urine when it was emptied before transfer from the recovery room. Carmen is awake and says she is "really tired." She received epidural morphine (Duramorph) prior to leaving the operating room and rates her pain as 0 on a pain scale. (Use information from Chapter 10 and also Chapters 7 and 9 to answer the questions in this exercise.)

   a. Identify the priority nursing diagnosis for Carmen during her recovery period. What interventions are appropriate for this nursing diagnosis? What other important nursing diagnosis should be considered? Why?

   b. Carmen's vital signs are: T 98.6, P 96, R 20, BP 110/90 1 hour later. Lochia is moderate, with some small clots. Her catheter bag contains a very small amount of urine. She is slightly restless, but says she has no pain. How should you interpret these assessments? What action should you take?

   c. Are other complications more likely to develop later in the postpartum period? What do you think they would be?

APPLYING KNOWLEDGE

1. Look at the graphic charts of several postpartum women. What is the pattern of their temperature and pulse rates after birth? Do you see any differences in these patterns among women who had a vaginal birth and those who had a cesarean birth?

2. Study the routine postpartum teaching given to all women before discharge. For each sign or symptom that a woman should report, identify the complications related to that sign or symptom.

3. Determine if your clinical facility provides written postpartum self-care instructions in languages other than English. If not, what provisions does the staff make for non-English–speaking patients?

Student Name_____

REVIEW QUESTIONS

(238, 241) **1.** A woman had a forceps-assisted birth 2 hours ago. Baseline vital signs were temperature 37.1° C (98.8° F), pulse 78, respirations 20, blood pressure 118/70. Which of the following assessments suggests possible development of hypovolemic shock?

1. firm fundus, slightly right of midline
2. pulse 100, respirations 24
3. respirations 22, blood pressure 114/76
4. light lochia rubra with small clots

(237-246) **2.** A woman had a 16-hour labor that ended with the cesarean birth of a 4313 g (9.5 lb) infant. Her membranes were ruptured for 24 hours and oxytocin augmentation of labor was attempted before the cesarean birth. She has an IV infusion of Ringers' lactate and an indwelling catheter. Which complication should the nurse be most observant for during the immediate recovery-room period?

1. uterine atony
2. endometritis
3. uterine subinvolution
4. urinary tract infection

(240-242) **3.** If the nurse finds that a new mother's uterus is soft, the appropriate initial action is to

1. insert an indwelling catheter.
2. massage the uterus until it is firm.
3. check the woman's vital signs.
4. increase the rate of the IV fluid.

(241-242) **4.** One hour after vaginal birth, the nurse notes that a woman has a flat purple area, about 2 cm by 3 cm, on her perineum. Which is the most appropriate nursing action at this time?

1. Assist her to take a warm sitz bath.
2. Apply pressure with a tightly applied pad.
3. Reapply a chemical cold pack on the area.
4. Notify the physician of the observation.

(247) **5.** When teaching a woman following vaginal birth 24 hours ago, the nurse should tell her to report

1. pink vaginal drainage followed by red drainage.
2. menstrual-like odor of vaginal discharge.
3. uterine cramping when the infant nurses.
4. excretion of large quantities of dilute urine.

(244) **6.** Choose the most appropriate intervention to prevent deep vein thrombosis in a woman who is one day postcesarean birth.

1. Encourage her to walk several times each day.
2. Provide her with increased fluids that she enjoys.
3. Take her temperature to identify an elevation.
4. Instruct her to stay in bed most of the day.

(244-245) **7.** Choose the finding that suggests infection after birth.

1. poorly relieved perineal pain 4 hours postpartum
2. oral temperature of 37.7° C (100° F) 18 hours postpartum
3. white blood cell count of 21,000/dl at 1 day postpartum
4. persistent and severe cramping 3 days postpartum

(245) **8.** The best position for the woman who has postpartum endometritis is

1. semi-sitting. 2. side-lying.
3. supine. 4. prone.

(245) **9.** Which nursing assessment suggests that a postpartum woman has cystitis?

1. burning with every urination
2. high fever accompanied by chills
3. fever with nausea and vomiting
4. voiding large amounts of urine

(245) **10.** Which nurse's teaching is appropriate for the new mother who has cystitis?

1. Eat several servings of whole grains and meats each day.
2. Remain in bed except for going to the bathroom.
3. Drink about 3 liters of noncaffeinated beverages daily.
4. Take a stool softener to reduce added pain of constipation.

(237-238) **11.** A woman is 8 hours postpartum after a spontaneous vaginal birth. Her admission hemoglobin was 10 g/dl, and her estimated blood loss during the birth was 750 ml. She asks the nurse if she can walk to the bathroom. The best nursing response is to

1. Remind her that she should catch her urine in a "hat" to be measured.
2. Have her sit briefly on the side of the bed before helping her to the bathroom.
3. Encourage her to urinate every 2 hours to decrease the risk of excess bleeding.
4. Tell her to return to bed promptly after she finishes using the bathroom.

(244-246) **12.** Which nursing assessment suggests infection of an episiotomy?

1. temperature of 38° C (100.4° F) 12 hours after birth
2. purplish discoloration of the perineum and labia
3. edema of the labia minora, labia majora, and perineum
4. redness of the perineum with separation of the suture line

(241) **13.** A woman has postpartum uterine atony with hemorrhage. After it is controlled, the physician orders an indwelling Foley catheter mainly because it

1. allows better estimation of the woman's blood volume.
2. identifies bloody urine that suggests bladder trauma.
3. limits the need for the woman to ambulate to the bathroom.
4. applies constant pressure against the bleeding uterus.

Student Name_____

(244-246) **14.** A woman who is 3 days postpartum comes to the emergency clinic because she is having pain and burning discomfort when she urinates. She denies that she has had any fever. The nurse should expect an initial order for

1. bladder analgesics.
2. intravenous antibiotics.
3. complete blood count.
4. clean-catch urine specimen.

(246-247) **15.** A woman is 5 days postpartum and breastfeeding. She telephones the nurse at the clinic and says that her breasts feel very heavy and one of them is tender. She says the infant nurses "fair." The nurse should tell the woman that

1. her symptoms should go away when the infant begins nursing better.
2. breastfeeding should be stopped until the pain goes away.
3. a cold pack between feedings should reduce the pain.
4. she should come to the clinic for evaluation of her symptoms.

(241) **16.** Methylergonovine (Methergine) should be avoided if the woman has

1. uterine atony.
2. retained placenta.
3. hypertension.
4. endometritis.

(242) **17.** Which of these postpartum women is at greatest risk for bleeding from a vaginal wall laceration?

1. She had a forceps-assisted vaginal birth.
2. She delivered a 3632 g (8 lb) infant.
3. She has a history of uterine atony.
4. Oxytocin (Pitocin) was used to induce labor.

(246) **18.** Choose the foods that are highest in iron.

1. citrus fruits, apricots, tomatoes
2. sweet and white potatoes, corn, dried beans
3. enriched bread, dark green leafy vegetables
4. milk, cheeses, legumes

(248) **19.** A woman comes to the clinic for her 6-week postpartum check after having her first baby. She says to the nurse, "I don't know what's wrong with me. I'm exhausted all the time and yet I can't seem to sleep when I have the chance." The nurse should

1. reassure her that the demands of being a mother can seem overwhelming, especially with the first baby.
2. ask her if her partner, family members, or friends can help her with care of the baby and her home so she can rest.
3. explain that women lose more blood at birth than they expect, and a slight anemia often leads to these symptoms.
4. find a quiet place to talk with her about her feelings related to her new role as a mother.

(249) **20.** Postpartum bipolar disorder is characterized by

1. periods of let-down feelings but with general enjoyment of life.
2. impaired reality characterized by euphoria alternating with depression.
3. alternate periods of overeating and lack of interest in food and drink.
4. prolonged feelings of worthlessness or guilt.

CHAPTER 11

The Nurse's Role in Women's Health Care

Answer Key: Textbook page references are provided as a guide for answering these questions. A complete answer key was provided for your instructor.

LEARNING ACTIVITIES

1. Match the terms in the left column with their definitions on the right (a–r).

(267)	_____ basal temperature	a. device inserted into vagina to support pelvic structures
(275)	_____ climacteric	b. painful sexual intercourse
(278-279)	_____ cystocele	c. presence of tissue resembling uterine lining outside the uterus
(255)	_____ dyspareunia	d. release of semen into the male's bladder during sexual intercourse
(255)	_____ endometriosis	e. stretching of the cervical mucus at ovulation
(269)	_____ infertility	f. body temperature at rest, taken before any activity
(276)	_____ libido	g. weak vaginal wall that cannot support the bladder properly
(275)	_____ menopause	h. weak posterior vaginal wall that inhibits proper stool passage
(271)	_____ myoma	i. inability to conceive when desired
(275, 276)	_____ osteoporosis	j. enlarged vein in the scrotum
(279)	_____ pessary	k. unexpected loss of urine when laughing, coughing, or sneezing
(279)	_____ rectocele	l. inability to control urge to urinate due to overactive bladder
(271)	_____ retrograde ejaculation	m. cessation of menstruation
(268)	_____ spinnbarkeit	n. benign tumors of the uterine muscle
(279)	_____ stress incontinence	o. sexual desire
(279)	_____ urge incontinence	p. period of time surrounding the cessation of menstruation
(279)	_____ uterine prolapse	q. loss of bone mass leading to bone fragility
(271)	_____ varicocele	r. weakened support ligaments for the vagina and uterus

(252)   **2.**   a.   The best time to perform breast self-examination is

_____ or

_____.

b.   Professional breast examination should be done _____ for all women over

the age of _____.

c.   The American Cancer Society recommends that mammography be done for all women

aged _____ at _____ intervals.

(252)   **3.**   List the preparation a woman should make before having a Pap test.

a.   _____

b.   _____

(253)   **4.**   a.   The Pap test is recommended at _____ intervals for all women age

_____ or older.

b.   Under what conditions can a Pap test be done less frequently?

_____

_____

(254-255) **5.**   Define each term that relates to menstrual disorders.

a.   Amenorrhea _____

b.   Primary amenorrhea _____

_____

c.   Secondary amenorrhea _____

_____

d.   Metrorrhagia _____

_____

e.   Menorrhagia _____

Student Name_____

f.   Mittelschmerz _____

_____

g.   Dysmenorrhea _____

_____

(254)   **6.**   How can a low body weight contribute to amenorrhea?

_____

_____

(255)   **7.**   List common symptoms of premenstrual dysphoric disorder (PMDD).

a.   _____

b.   _____

c.   _____

d.   _____

e.   _____

f.   _____

g.   _____

h.   _____

i.   _____

j.   _____

k.   _____

(255)   **8.**   a.   When do the symptoms of PMDD occur?

_____

b.   How many of the typical symptoms are required to diagnose PMDD?

_____

c.   Describe therapy that may be prescribed for PMDD. _____

_____

_____

d.   Explain nursing responsibilities related to PMDD. _____

_____

(256)   **9.**   List four factors that contribute to vaginal infection and why they increase this risk.

a.   _____

b.   _____

c.   _____

d.   _____

(256)   **10.**   Describe important teaching related to toxic shock syndrome in each area listed.

a.   Hand washing

_____

_____

b.   Use of tampons

_____

_____

c.   Use of cervical cap or diaphragm for contraception

_____

_____

(258)   **11.**   a.   Describe signs and symptoms of candidiasis.

_____

_____

b.   List common medications used to treat candidiasis.

_____

_____

(257, 260) **12.**   a.   What is the most prevalent viral sexually transmissible infection?

_____

Student Name _____

b.   What are the characteristics of this infection?

_____

_____

c.   What complications may occur during birth or after birth for the infant?

_____

d.   What malignant complication is associated with the infection and what precautions should the woman take related to this associated complication?

_____

_____

(257-258) **13.** How can infections of Chlamydia or gonorrhea result in infertility or an ectopic pregnancy?

_____

_____

(257, 259) **14.** a.   The STD that has three possible stages is _____.

b.   Describe the characteristics of each stage of this infection.

Primary _____

_____

Secondary_____

_____

Tertiary_____

_____

c.   What is the main drug used to treat it? Which alternate drug must be avoided during pregnancy? _____

_____

(257, 259) **15.** Infections of _____ can reemerge later in outbreaks that are

also infectious.

(262)   **16.** a.   Most oral contraceptives contain _____ and

_____, while some contain only _____.

b.   How does this drug or combination of drugs prevent pregnancy?

_____

(262-263) **17.** What is the significance of the ACHES acronym in relation to oral contraceptives? What does each letter stand for?

_____

_____

_____

_____

_____

_____

(263-264) **18.** Depo-Provera provides _____ months of effective contraception. It is given by the

_____ route within _____ days of the menstrual period. Why is this timing

important?

(264)   **19.** List the three most common side effects of Depo-Provera.

a.   _____

b.   _____

c.   _____

(264)   **20.** What is the major difference among these intrauterine devices in terms of effectiveness?

a.   Copper-containing (ParaGard) _____

b.   Levonorgestrel-releasing _____

c.   Progesterone-releasing _____

(264-265) **21.** List two times when the diaphragm must be refitted.

a.   _____

b.   _____

(265-266) **22.** Describe appropriate teaching about condom use in each area listed.

a.   Lubrication _____

_____

Student Name_____

    b.   Breakage or dislodgment during use _____

    _____

    c.   Expiration date_____

    d.   Removal _____

    _____

(267-268) **23.** Describe three methods that can be used for natural family planning.

    a.   _____

    _____

    b.   _____

    _____

    c.   _____

    _____

(268-269) **24.** Why must another form of contraception be used for about 1 month following vasectomy?

    _____

    _____

(269) **25.** Describe four types of emergency contraception, including administration.

    a.   Oral contraceptives or Preven kit_____

    _____

    b.   Levonorgestrel _____

    _____

    c.   Intrauterine device_____

    _____

    d.   Mifepristone (RU 486)_____

    _____

(269-270) **26.** a.   Define *primary infertility.*

    _____

b.   Define *secondary infertility*.

_____

(270)   **27.**   Describe the psychological reactions a couple may have to infertility.

_____

_____

_____

_____

_____

(270-272) **28.**   a.   Describe how each male factor can compromise fertility.

Abnormal sperm _____

_____

Abnormal erections _____

_____

Abnormal ejaculation _____

_____

Abnormal seminal fluid _____

_____

b.   Describe how each female factor can compromise fertility.

Disorders of ovulation _____

_____

Abnormalities of fallopian tubes _____

_____

Abnormalities of uterus, cervix, or ovaries _____

_____

Hormone abnormalities_____

_____

Student Name_____

(273-274) **29.** Describe similarities and differences among the following assisted reproductive techniques.

    a.   In vitro fertilization (IVF) _____

        _____

    b.   Gamete intrafallopian transfer (GIFT) _____

        _____

    c.   Tubal embryo transfer (TET)_____

        _____

    d.   Microsurgery _____

        _____

(275-276) **30.** Describe the following changes that may occur during the climacteric.

    a.   Menstrual cycles_____

        _____

    b.   Vasomotor instability_____

        _____

(276) **31.** Describe changes in these structures that occur with loss of estrogen.

    a.   Uterus and ovaries _____

        _____

    b.   Vagina _____

        _____

    c.   Pelvic musculature _____

        _____

    d.   Bones _____

        _____

(274-275) **32.** a.   Describe the major advantages of hormone replacement therapy (HRT).

        _____

        _____

b.   Explain conditions in which HRT is contraindicated.

_____

_____

(275)   **33.** List five types of complementary therapy that may be used instead of, or as an alternative to, HRT and the purpose for each.

a.   _____

b.   _____

c.   _____

d.   _____

e.   _____

(279)   **34.** Describe each variation of vaginal wall prolapse.

a.   Cystocele _____

_____

b.   Rectocele _____

_____

(280)   **35.** What treatments may be used to reduce symptomatic uterine myomas?

a.   Medical treatment _____

_____

_____

b.   Surgical treatment _____

_____

_____

THINKING CRITICALLY

1.   When in your orthopedic experience, note how many women are affected with hip fractures compared to the number of men affected. Does one ethnic group seem to be more affected than others? Do you notice signs of osteoporosis in these patients?

Student Name_____

APPLYING KNOWLEDGE

1. Interview nurses at a clinic about their experience caring for patients with STDs. Which diseases are most prevalent?

2. Under supervision, teach a woman to perform a breast self-examination (BSE).

REVIEW QUESTIONS

(252-253) 1. The nurse is teaching a woman, age 25, about BSE. The correct teaching is that BSE
1. detects malignancy more often than professional examinations.
2. allows her to delay the need for mammography until she is 50 years old.
3. helps her learn the normal characteristics of her own breasts.
4. is more accurate than a yearly mammogram.

(252-253) 2. Choose the correct teaching about BSE technique.
1. Use the palms of the hand to press the breast tissue firmly against the ribs.
2. Palpate each breast systematically, using the pads of the fingers.
3. Palpate the underarm area only if the breasts are very large and sagging.
4. Squeeze the breast tissue between the thumb and index finger.

(255) 3. Choose the correct teaching for relief of symptoms associated with premenstrual dysphoric syndrome.
1. Eat chocolate candies several times a day to reduce fluid retention and weight gain.
2. Reduce fluid intake during the first half of the menstrual cycle.
3. Plan the most stressful activities during the last half of the menstrual cycle.
4. Exercise individually or with others several times each week.

(256) 4. When teaching about the use of tampons, the nurse should emphasize replacing them at least every 4 hours to prevent
1. pelvic inflammatory disease.
2. vasomotor symptoms.
3. sexually transmissible disease.
4. toxic shock syndrome.

(258) 5. A friend asks you what she can do because she is troubled by repeated "yeast" infections. As a nurse, your best advice to her is to
1. keep over-the-counter medications on hand so she can begin treatment immediately.
2. see her medical caregiver if she has another infection to identify possible causes.
3. increase her intake of fluids to include at least eight glasses of water each day.
4. avoid sexual intercourse for 1 month to see if that reduces the infections.

(257, 260) 6. The long-term risk of an infection with the human papillomavirus is for
1. cervical cancer.
2. ectopic pregnancy.
3. endometriosis.
4. nerve damage.

(261, 265) 7. Other than abstinence, the best way to prevent sexually transmitted infection with the human immunodeficiency virus is

1. douching within 30 minutes of sexual intercourse.
2. avoiding intercourse during midcycle.
3. use of a condom for all episodes of sexual intercourse.
4. taking prophylactic antibiotics after unprotected intercourse.

(262) 8. Choose the most appropriate teaching for the woman who is prescribed multiphasic oral contraceptive pills.

1. The menstrual period begins when the 4th week of pills is completed.
2. Cigarette smoking should be limited to no more than 10 per day.
3. Limit intake of foods that are high in iron or calcium.
4. Take the pills at the same time of day and in order.

(262) 9. Choose the woman who should not take oral contraceptives.

1. A woman who has multiple sexual partners.
2. A 38-year-old woman who smokes a pack of cigarettes daily.
3. A 19-year-old woman who is formula feeding her 2-month-old baby.
4. A woman who is being discharged after a spontaneous abortion.

(262) 10. A woman has been taking oral contraceptives for 4 months. She is concerned because her periods are much lighter than before she started the pills. How should the nurse counsel this woman?

1. "You will probably have to discontinue the pill unless your periods become more like they were previously."
2. "We can switch you to a barrier contraceptive; your periods should return to normal in just a few months."
3. "Lighter periods are expected when you are on the pill but you should tell us if they stop entirely."
4. "Stop taking the pills immediately. We want to do a pregnancy test before you resume them."

(264) 11. Choose the correct patient teaching about the IUD.

1. "You should not use this contraception if you smoke or are over 35."
2. "Check for the strings weekly for the first 4 weeks, then monthly."
3. "Do not use tampons when you have your menstrual period."
4. "Use another form of contraception for the first month after insertion."

(265) 12. Choose the contraceptive method from those listed that provides the best protection against sexually transmitted diseases.

1. female condom
2. hormone injection
3. intrauterine device
4. oral contraceptives

(268) **13.** When teaching a woman the cervical mucus method to identify ovulation, the nurse teaches her that the normal character of the mucus near ovulation is

   1. slippery and stretchy.
   2. yellowish with a distinct odor.
   3. cloudy and sticky.
   4. thick, sticky, and clear.

(268-269) **14.** Appropriate patient teaching following vasectomy is to

   1. apply heat to the operative area for 20 minutes at a time.
   2. abstain from intercourse for at least 6 weeks after the surgery.
   3. limit frequency of sexual intercourse for the first month.
   4. place an ice pack on the operative area to reduce discomfort.

(276) **15.** A friend tells you that she is "having periods again." She thought she had her last menstrual period 2 years ago. As a nurse, you should advise her that she

   1. is probably having reactivation of estrogens that are causing the bleeding.
   2. should see a physician promptly because this is not an expected occurrence.
   3. may be ovulating again and should use a contraceptive if she does not want to become pregnant.
   4. probably has an infection of her vagina or cervix that should be treated to prevent further infection.

(276, 277) **16.** "Hot flashes" are probably caused by

   1. anxiety about growing older and one's mortality.
   2. shifts in a woman's fluid and electrolyte balance.
   3. instability of the blood pressure.
   4. reduced estrogen secretion.

(275) **17.** Choose the correct patient teaching about the drug alendronate (Fosamax).

   1. Take food or milk within 30 minutes of the medication.
   2. Wash the nose out with saline 30 minutes after using the spray.
   3. Do not lie down for at least 30 minutes after taking the drug.
   4. Take calcium supplements at the same time as the medication.

(279) **18.** Stress incontinence is best described as loss of urine

   1. during activities such as laughing or coughing.
   2. when in an anxiety-provoking situation.
   3. when vaginal infection occurs.
   4. during sexual intercourse.

(280) **19.** What is the usual diagnostic procedure when an ovarian cyst is suspected?

   1. transvaginal ultrasound examination
   2. bimanual pelvic examination
   3. laparotomy with biopsy
   4. magnetic resonance image

(279) **20.** A nursing measure that can improve stress incontinence is to

   1. teach the woman to limit fluid intake to eight glasses of water each day.
   2. advise her to increase her fiber intake with raw vegetables and fruits and whole grains.
   3. encourage weight-bearing exercise at least three times each week.
   4. explain how and when to perform the Kegel exercises.

CHAPTER

12

Student Name _____

The Term Newborn

Answer Key: Textbook page references are provided as a guide for answering these questions. A complete answer key was provided for your instructor.

LEARNING ACTIVITIES

(282)   **1.**   Why is it important that a governmental agency collect statistical information about births and deaths in the neonatal and infant periods of life?

_____

_____

(283-284) **2.**   Describe each reflex and state the age at which it is expected to disappear.

Reflex	Description	Age at Disappearance
Moro		
Rooting		
Tonic neck		
Dancing		

(284)   **3.**   Normal newborn head circumference ranges from _____ inches to _____

inches, or from _____ cm to _____ cm.

(284-285) **4.**   List two functions of an infant's fontanels.

a.   _____

_____

b.   _____

_____

(285)   **5.**   Describe the following characteristics of the anterior fontanel.

a.   Shape _____

b.   Location (bones) _____

c.   Time of closure _____

(285)   **6.**   Describe the following characteristics of the posterior fontanel.

a.   Shape _____

b.   Location (bones) _____

c.   Time of closure _____

(288)   **7.**   Describe the three steps for using a bulb suction to remove excess secretions.

a.   _____

b.   _____

c.   _____

(288)   **8.**   Explain the two types of heart murmurs that can be heard in newborns. Indicate which may
cause problems.

a.   Functional _____

_____

b.   Organic _____

_____

Student Name_____

(289) **9.** a. What is a common route for taking a newborn's first temperature?

_____

b. Subsequent temperatures are taken by what route?

_____

c. What is the correct technique for taking the temperature by each method?

_____

_____

(289-290) **10.** State normal ranges for each of these newborn vital signs and signs that the nurse should promptly report.

Vital Sign	Normal Range (state both Fahrenheit and centigrade)	Signs to Report (include both rate and character as appropriate)
Temperature		
Pulse		
Respirations		

(290) **11.** Give the average range for these newborn measurements.

a. Length _____ to _____ inches (_____ to _____ cm)

b. Weight _____ to _____ pounds (_____ to _____ g)

(290) **12.** Describe the following normal musculoskeletal assessments for a newborn, including possible deviations from normal.

a. Movements_____

b. Eyes _____

_____

124   Study Guide to accompany Introduction to Maternity & Pediatric Nursing, Fourth Edition

    c.   Tremors _____

    _____

    d.   Muscle tone _____

    _____

(291)   **13.**   Describe the following characteristics and functions of a newborn infant's kidneys.

    a.   Blood flow _____

    _____

    b.   Reabsorption functions _____

    _____

    c.   Concentration of urine _____

    _____

    d.   Capacity to handle fluid imbalances _____

    _____

(291-292) **14.**   Expectant parents are attending a prepared childbirth class in which you discuss circumcision. Several ask you if their sons should have the procedure done and another couple said they thought all boys were circumcised. What should you tell these couples about the advantages and disadvantages of circumcision. What should you tell them about circumcision in the Jewish faith?

    a.   Advantages _____

    _____

    b.   Disadvantages _____

    _____

    c.   Circumcision in Jewish families _____

    _____

(292)   **15.**   Explain each of the following aspects of circumcision care in a way you might teach parents.

    a.   Pain relief that may be used _____

    _____

Student Name_____

        b.   Comforting _____

_____

        c.   Maintaining warmth _____

_____

        c.   Bleeding _____

_____

        d.   Urination _____

_____

(295)   **16.** Explain the normal occurrences that cause physiologic jaundice.

_____

_____

_____

(295)   **17.** a.   Physiologic jaundice appears at about _____ days after birth and lasts for

                about _____ days.

        b.   Pathologic jaundice may appear within _____ day(s) after birth.

(295)   **18.** Describe the following typical stools in the newborn, including the time they appear, if applicable.

        a.   Meconium _____

_____

        b.   Transitional stool _____

_____

        c.   Stool of breastfed baby _____

_____

        d.   Stool of formula-fed baby _____

_____

(295)   **19.**   Describe three types of abnormal stools in the newborn.

a. _____

b. _____

c. _____

(297)   **20.**   Describe stools in constipation.

_____

_____

(297)   **21.**   The newborn's stomach has a capacity of about _____ ml and empties in about

_____ hours.

(297)   **22.**   Why is it important to prevent infection in a newborn and what characteristic of the newborn's response to infection can make it difficult to recognize?

_____

_____

CASE STUDY

1.   Sandra and Jim Black, a couple in their mid-20s, have a new baby son named Justin who is now 16 hours old, weighs 7 pounds, 9 ounces, and is breastfeeding. Sandra wants to go home about 36 hours after birth. Justin will be circumcised (Plastibell) before discharge. Sandra and Jim have no nearby relatives and are the first couple in their circle of friends to have a baby. They have read books on baby care, but are concerned about actually caring for their baby's needs. Sandra and Jim say they need to know "everything." For each area listed, explain what content you will teach them. How can you encourage the parents to participate in each topic so they will feel more secure? How will you incorporate information they may have read in books? You are encouraged to incorporate any of your facility's teaching materials as you complete this case study.

a.   Safety

b.   Using bulb syringe

c.   Taking their baby's temperature

d.   Maintaining an optimal body temperature

2.   Because Justin will be discharged soon after being circumcised, what should you teach the parents about care and observation for complications? What actions may comfort him?

Student Name _____

APPLYING KNOWLEDGE

1. Assist with admitting newborns after birth. Administer prophylactic eye care and vitamin K injections. What initial and ongoing cord care does your facility use? Does your facility offer the first hepatitis B immunization with newborn care? Do parents sign a consent form for any of these procedures? Which one(s)?

2. Observe newborns in the nursery for characteristics listed in the textbook. Distinguish between normal characteristics and those that may indicate a problem. What action is taken for deviations from normal?

3. Observe a circumcision. What type of circumcision is most common in your hospital? Observe newborns after circumcision for bleeding and urination.

4. Does your hospital have a standard infant care teaching plan for new parents? If so, what does the plan include? Observe how different staff nurses incorporate parent teaching into their care of mothers and babies. How have short stays influenced parent teaching?

5. A new baby is coming to the office for a checkup at 1 week of age. He weighed 8 pounds, 6 ounces at birth. He now weighs 7 pounds, 7 ounces. Has the baby's weight loss been within normal limits or is it excessive? Justify your answer.

REVIEW QUESTIONS

(283) 1. Which reflex shows the baby's reaction to sudden movement by drawing up the legs, extending the arms, then folding the arms across the chest with the fingers open?

1. dancing 2. Moro
3. rooting 4. grasp

(283) 2. When teaching a mother how to nurse her baby, how should you explain the baby's rooting reflex? The rooting reflex

1. shows equality of function on each side of the mouth.
2. helps the baby keep mucus or milk from being inhaled during breathing.
3. suggests that the baby is full as he or she turns away from the breast.
4. is the baby's way of seeking her nipple to obtain milk when hungry.

(283-284) 3. In the birthing room, a first-time father asks the nurse why the baby's head is "long and pointy." The nurse should respond

1. "The head changes shape so it can pass through the mother's pelvis during birth."
2. "Fluid builds up within the head before and during birth; it will go away in a few days."
3. "Labor causes slight bleeding into the space between the skull bones and their covering."
4. "We will notify the pediatrician, who will probably order an MRI of the baby's head."

(286) 4. Visually, babies prefer

1. geometric objects.
2. soft or pastel colors.
3. the human face.
4. stationary objects.

(288)   5.   The correct way to suction a baby's mouth with a bulb syringe is to

1.   compress the bulb, place the tip in the side of the mouth, then release the bulb.
2.   place the tip in the side of the mouth, compress the bulb, then release the bulb.
3.   compress the bulb, place the tip in the center of the mouth, then release the bulb.
4.   place the tip in the center of the mouth, compress the bulb, then release the bulb.

(289)   6.   When admitted to the nursery, a baby's initial rectal temperature is 96.6° F (35.8° C). Choose the most appropriate nursing response for this assessment.

1.   Chart the expected temperature and continue doing other admission assessments and measurements.
2.   Keep the baby in a radiant warmer during admission and recheck the temperature in 30 minutes.
3.   Remove blankets and sources of added heat from the baby.
4.   Recheck the temperature in 30 minutes to verify accuracy.

(292)   7.   One hour after a Plastibell circumcision, the nurse notes a small amount of blood oozing from the area. Which is the appropriate initial nursing response to this observation?

1.   Continue to observe for increased bleeding.
2.   Apply pressure with a gauze pad and gloved fingers.
3.   Call the physician who performed the procedure.
4.   Wrap petroleum jelly gauze around the penis.

(295)   8.   A new mother asks why her 2-day-old baby's skin appears slightly yellow. Which is the best nursing response to explain the cause of this skin color?

1.   Small blood vessels are broken during labor, releasing waste products into the blood.
2.   The baby's digestive tract is immature and cannot yet excrete bilirubin effectively.
3.   Skin color changes slightly during the first few weeks until the permanent color is evident.
4.   Excess blood cells are being broken down rapidly because the baby is now breathing air.

(295)   9.   New parents should be taught to clean their baby's ears by

1.   moistening a cotton-tipped applicator with water and rotating it in the ear canal.
2.   gently instilling a small amount of warm water into the ear with a bulb syringe.
3.   applying baby oil to a rolled piece of cotton and inserting it into the ear.
4.   wiping the outside with cotton that is moistened with water.

(295)   10.   A small area of a term infant's abdominal skin remains distorted when pinched gently. This assessment suggests

1.   poor hydration.
2.   postbirth edema.
3.   excessive intake of breast milk or formula.
4.   inadequate vernix during the prenatal period.

Student Name _____

(295, 297) **11.** What should the parents be taught about caring for the umbilical cord?

1. Bathe the baby in a small basin to cleanse the cord on all surfaces.
2. A sponge bath is easy and allows the cord to remain dry until healed.
3. Use an oil-based cleanser to speed healing of the baby's cord site.
4. Baths are not needed until the cord site has healed to reduce infection.

(297) **12.** An infant has a small laceration on the forehead when delivered by cesarean. Brief finger pressure in the operating room stopped the bleeding and the physician does not need to suture the laceration. The nurse should primarily observe for what other complication related to the baby's laceration?

1. anemia, possibly manifested by pallor and tachycardia
2. hypothermia due to delay of placement in a warmer
3. excessive erythrocyte destruction and early jaundice
4. infection limited to the site or possibly generalized

(287, 292) **13.** A newborn has a heelstick for studies. The mother is concerned because the baby is crying loudly. The best response of the nurse is

1. "That's the only way the baby can communicate with us."
2. "Hold the baby close and comfort him by gentle rocking."
3. "Babies cannot feel pain because they are immature."
4. "The baby will only cry for a few minutes at most."

(292) **14.** How should the nurse respond to acrocyanosis in a 12-hour-old infant?

1. Administer oxygen through an infant-sized mask.
2. Apply heat with an incubator or radiant warmer.
3. Assess the pulse and respirations for abnormal rates.
4. Continue routine newborn nursing observations.

(290) **15.** Which is an abnormal assessment for a Latino boy at 5 days of age? Birth weight was 8 pounds, 5 ounces (3772 g); vital signs on discharge from the hospital were: T 98.4° F (axillary); P 142; R 40. There were no complications during pregnancy.

1. The infant weighs 7 pounds, 5 ounces (3318 g).
2. The apical pulse is 130/bpm and slightly irregular.
3. The infant has bluish areas on the lower back.
4. The infant has tiny white raised papules on the nose.

(290) **16.** A new mother asks why her term newborn sometimes "shakes" when he cries. Choose the best nursing response.

1. "Why not ask the baby's doctor about this when she makes rounds?"
2. "The baby is easily upset and waves his arms to show his irritation."
3. "An infant's muscles are too weak to move steadily."
4. "This is a normal newborn behavior during crying."

(295) **17.** A term newborn should pass the first meconium stool no later than how many hours after birth?

1. 6
2. 12
3. 24
4. 36

(292)   **18.** A new mother is concerned because her 3-day-old daughter has a slightly blood-tinged vaginal mucus discharge. How should the nurse respond to this mother's concern?

1. "The baby could have a minor abnormality in her vagina."
2. "Has there been any kind of injury to this area?"
3. "Effects of your pregnancy hormones cause this response."
4. "This should be reported to the doctor right away."

(295)   **19.** The nurse should teach parents to avoid using baby powder because it

1. irritates the respiratory tract.
2. may cause allergies in the newborn.
3. is difficult to remove during a bath.
4. dries the skin of the axillae and groin.

(287)   **20.** An infant looks at her mother and remains quiet when the mother sings to her in soft, high-pitched tones. This is an example of

1. a sign of impaired hearing.
2. the quiet alert state of reactivity.
3. a need for reduced stimulation.
4. limited ability to respond to adults.

Student Name_____

● **CROSSWORD PUZZLE**

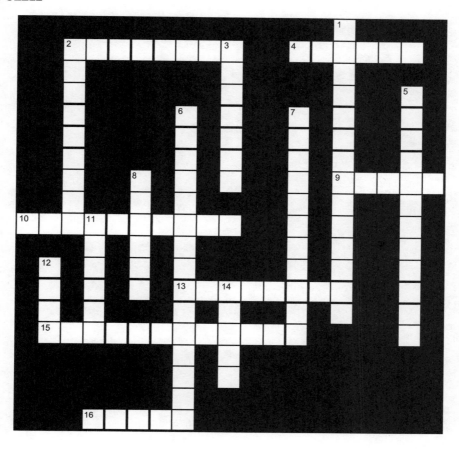

Across

(295)	2.	First stool
(292)	4.	Fetal skin protectant from watery environment
(284)	9.	Edema of the scalp
(284-285)	10.	Soft area at intersection of skull bones
(292)	13.	Pearl-type white dots on the hard palate
(292)	15.	Bluish color to the hands and/or feet
(292)	16.	Small white bumps, usually on the nose or chin

Down

(291)	1.	Failure of the testes to descend into the scrotum
(292)	2.	Bluish spots or discolorations of the skin, usually in dark-skinned babies
(283-284)	3.	Shaping of the head from pressure during birth
(291)	5.	Removal of the foreskin of the penis
(284)	6.	Collection of blood beneath the periosteum of the skull
(291)	7.	Urethral opening on underside of penis
(292)	8.	Fine hair covering the body
(295)	11.	Term used to describe the amount of tissue elasticity
(292)	12.	Topical anesthetic used for pain relief during circumcision
(292)	14.	"Bites" that are not really bites, but reddish areas on the back of the neck and eyelids

CHAPTER

13 Preterm and Postterm Newborns

Answer Key: Textbook page references are provided as a guide for answering these questions. A complete answer key was provided for your instructor.

LEARNING ACTIVITIES

1. Match the terms in the left column with their definitions on the right (a–p).

(309)	_____ apnea	a. provision of full nutrition by the parenteral (IV) route
(306-307)	_____ Ballard	b. length of time spent in the uterus
(310)	_____ bradycardia	c. cessation of breathing for 20 seconds or more
(309)	_____ bronchopulmonary dysplasia	d. lung secretion that facilitates oxygen exchange
(313)	_____ circadian rhythm	e. nervous system damage caused by high levels of bilirubin in the blood
(305)	_____ gestational age	f. method of estimating newborn maturity by physical and neurological characteristics
(310)	_____ hypoglycemia	g. heart rate lower than 100 beats/min in the newborn
(314)	_____ kangaroo care	h. generalized infection
(312)	_____ kernicterus	i. low blood glucose (blood sugar) level
(313)	_____ neutral thermal environment	j. control of temperature, air, surface temperature, and humidity to minimize an infant's oxygen consumption
(306)	_____ preterm gestation	k. less than 38 weeks of gestation
(306)	_____ postterm gestation	l. 38 to 42 weeks of gestation
(310)	_____ sepsis	m. more than 42 weeks of gestation
(308)	_____ surfactant	n. warming an infant by skin-to-skin contact
(306)	_____ term gestation	o. sleep pattern
(314)	_____ total parenteral nutrition	p. condition that may cause an infant to have a prolonged dependence on a ventilator

(306)   **2.**   Describe the following typical physical characteristics of a preterm infant's appearance.

    a.   Skin _____

    b.   Superficial veins _____

    c.   Subcutaneous fat _____

    d.   Lanugo _____

    e.   Vernix caseosa _____

    f.   Sole creases _____

    g.   Abdomen _____

    h.   Nails _____

    i.   Genitalia _____

(308-309)   **3.**   a.   Respiratory distress syndrome (RDS) is associated with an inadequate quantity of

        _____ in the lungs.

    b.   At what gestation is an infant expected to have an adequate quantity of this substance?

        _____

    c.   If an infant is born before the gestation in 3 b, what is the usual therapy?

        _____

(309)   **4.**   If preterm birth appears inevitable, what drug for the mother should the nurse anticipate before birth?

    _____

(309-310)   **5.**   List two signs that may accompany apnea.

    a.   _____

    b.   _____

(310)   **6.**   List seven factors that make the preterm infant more vulnerable to loss of body heat than a term infant.

    a.   _____

    b.   _____

    c.   _____

Student Name_____

    d.   _____

    e.   _____

    f.   _____

    g.   _____

(310)   **7.**   a.   *Hypoglycemia* in the infant is defined as a plasma level of glucose lower than

          _____ mg/dl.

    b.   List two reasons why a preterm infant is prone to hypoglycemia.

        _____

        _____

(311)   **8.**   What two factors predispose a preterm infant to bleeding?

    a.   _____

    b.   _____

(312)   **9.**   Describe five factors that impair the preterm infant's nutritional function.

    a.   _____

    b.   _____

    c.   _____

    d.   _____

    e.   _____

(312)   **10.**   a.   What is the pathology of necrotizing enterocolitis (NEC)?

        _____

        _____

    b.   List signs that an infant may have NEC.

        _____

        _____

(312)   **11.** a.   For physiologic jaundice the upper limit of bilirubin concentration is _____

mg/dl in the term infant and _____ mg/dl in the preterm infant.

b.   Pathologic jaundice may appear within _____ (time) and/or may increase

at a rate greater than _____/24 hours.

c.   Breast milk jaundice usually appears at _____ (time) and rises no higher than

_____ /24 hours.

(314)   **12.** The ideal milk for the preterm infant is _____ milk.

(314)   **13.** List three methods by which the preterm infant can receive nourishment.

a.   _____

b.   _____

c.   _____

(314)   **14.** a.   The two usual positions for the preterm infant are _____ or

_____.

b.   What two alternate positions may be used for the preterm infant and why?

_____

_____

(318)   **15.** List seven problems that are associated with caring for a postterm newborn.

a.   _____

b.   _____

c.   _____

d.   _____

e.   _____

f.   _____

g.   _____

Student Name _____

(318)   **16.**   Describe the following typical physical characteristics of the postterm newborn.

a.   General body appearance _____

_____

b.   Presence of lanugo _____

_____

c.   Presence of vernix caseosa _____

_____

d.   Skin appearance _____

_____

THINKING CRITICALLY

1.   A friend had her baby at 32 weeks gestation 6 months ago. She confides that she is afraid her baby is not normal because he does not do the same things her first baby (born full-term) did at 6 months old. What can you tell your friend to reassure her?

APPLYING KNOWLEDGE

1.   Observe newborns of different gestational ages in your clinical facility. Identify differences in these characteristics. Determine whether the mother's "due date" correlates with the physical characteristics you see.
a.   Head and body hair
b.   Body posture and muscle tone
c.   Stiffness of ear cartilage
d.   Amount of breast tissue
e.   Appearance of genitalia
f.   Number and depth of sole creases

2.   Observe different methods of feeding preterm infants. What precautions are taken to ensure that the baby receives adequate nutrition without overload?

3.   If your facility does not routinely care for sick newborns, does it have arrangements with a larger hospital to transport these babies to a special care nursery? What is involved in transporting a sick baby? When do most newborns return to the original facility?

4.   How does your facility foster parent-infant bonding when an infant is sick or preterm? Is kangaroo care used?

5.   What treatment is used for jaundice that exceeds safe limits in your facility? Look up the protocols for nursing care that accompany this treatment.

REVIEW QUESTIONS

(306, 307) **1.** Which of the following physical characteristics should make the nurse think an infant's gestational age may be preterm?

    1. square window sign assessed at 0 degrees
    2. small amount of lanugo and vernix present
    3. labia majora cover labia minora of the female
    4. superficial scalp and abdominal veins easily seen

(306, 307) **2.** Gestational age is best determined with

    1. weight of the infant at birth.
    2. stability of the blood glucose level.
    3. the rate at which the infant reaches developmental milestones.
    4. assessment of physical and neurological characteristics.

(310) **3.** A preterm infant is subject to hypothermia because the

    1. muscle activity is large related to the calories consumed.
    2. relatively large body surface area allows heat to escape.
    3. sweat glands are overactive, allowing evaporative cooling.
    4. fat stores insulate the infant from radiant heater warmth.

(310) **4.** Choose the normal blood glucose level for a preterm infant.

    1. 28 mg/dl   2.   39 mg/dl
    3. 55 mg/dl   4.   150 mg/dl

(311) **5.** The nurse must handle the preterm infant gently because capillaries are

    1. not developed in all areas of the brain.
    2. likely to develop microscopic clots.
    3. sensitive to high levels of clotting factors.
    4. fragile and prone to bleed spontaneously.

(314) **6.** The advantage of radiant heaters in the care of preterm infants is that they

    1. cannot cause excessive body temperature.
    2. maintain warmth with easy caregiver access.
    3. reduce drying and cracking of the skin.
    4. improve balance of fluids and electrolytes.

(314) **7.** The ideal feeding for most preterm newborns is

    1. glucose water until the risk for necrotizing enterocolitis diminishes.
    2. breast milk given by suckling, bottle, or gavage.
    3. special commercial formula for preterm babies.
    4. total parenteral nutrition to meet all the infant's nutritional needs.

(318) **8.** An infant is brought to the newborn nursery. The gestation stated on the chart is 39 weeks. The nurse doing the initial assessment notes that the infant has peeling skin and a long, thin appearance. What is the probable reason for the infant's appearance?

    1. The mother did not get adequate nutrients throughout pregnancy.
    2. Intrauterine infection depleted subcutaneous fat stores.
    3. The actual gestational age may be greater than 42 weeks.
    4. Reduced production of glucose before birth caused weight loss.

Student Name_____

(317) **9.** A mother gives birth to a preterm infant at 30 weeks gestation. When visiting the baby in the intensive care unit, she seems interested in the baby, but sits and watches everything the nurse does for her baby. Which is the most appropriate nursing intervention to promote mother-infant attachment?

1. Invite her to provide simple care to her infant.
2. Reassure her that she can hold the baby soon.
3. Stress the importance of frequent visits to the nursery.
4. Demonstrate the skills she will need for home care.

(308) **10.** Which nursing assessment best suggests respiratory distress syndrome?

1. apical heart rate 144/min; bluish hands and feet
2. grunting, respiratory rate of 65/min, nasal flaring
3. protruding abdomen, irregular respirations
4. weak movements, lies with extended posture

(309-310) **11.** The alarm on an apnea monitor for a preterm infant sounds. The infant is asleep, the skin color is pink, and the heart rate is 130–135/min. The most appropriate initial nursing response is to

1. contact the physician for orders.
2. gently rub the infant's back.
3. give oxygen with an Ambu bag.
4. suction the infant with a bulb syringe.

(311) **12.** A key nursing intervention to prevent retinopathy of prematurity is to

1. provide feedings as early as possible after birth.
2. perform care to avoid moving the infant more than necessary.
3. eliminate potential sources of infection from the environment.
4. monitor the infant's blood oxygen levels.

(317-318) **13.** Most problems of the postterm infant result from

1. decreased functioning of the placenta.
2. reduced blood clotting factors.
3. increased susceptibility to infection.
4. increased subcutaneous fat deposits.

(312-313) **14.** Choose the bilirubin level or levels that should be reported to the physician for an infant of 38 weeks gestation.

1. 4 mg/dl at 18 hours after birth; 12 mg prior to discharge at 36 hours
2. 6 mg/dl at 24 hours after birth; sclerae and face are yellowish
3. 9 mg/dl prior to hospital discharge at 48 hours after birth
4. 6 mg/dl at 24 hours after birth; infant is breastfeeding well

CHAPTER 14

The Newborn with a Congenital Malformation

Answer Key: Textbook page references are provided as a guide for answering these questions. A complete answer key was provided for your instructor.

LEARNING ACTIVITIES

1. Match the terms in the left column with their definitions on the right (a–o).

(327)	_____ cheiloplasty	a.	inspection of a cavity or organ by passing a light through its walls
(325)	_____ habilitation	b.	suggests developmental hip dysplasia
(321)	_____ hydrocephalus	c.	teaching a skill to a child who is handicapped from birth
(340)	_____ hyperbilirubinemia	d.	maintains hip abduction in the treatment of developmental hip dysplasia
(340)	_____ kernicterus	e.	single transverse line across the palm
(344)	_____ macrosomia	f.	brain damage due to accumulation of bilirubin in the brain tissue
(324)	_____ meningocele	g.	large fetal or newborn body size
(324)	_____ myelodysplasia	h.	surgical repair of a cleft lip
(324)	_____ myelomeningocele	i.	partial displacement of the head of the femur from the acetabulum
(331)	_____ Ortolani's sign	j.	excess blood levels of bilirubin
(331)	_____ Pavlik harness	k.	presence of three chromosomes in a body cell
(337)	_____ simian crease	l.	group of malformations of the spinal cord
(330-331)	_____ subluxation	m.	accumulation of cerebrospinal fluid within the brain's ventricles
(321)	_____ transillumination	n.	form of spina bifida in which portions of the membranes and cerebrospinal fluid are contained in a cystic mass
(337)	_____ trisomy	o.	form of spina bifida that consists of protrusion of a saclike cyst containing meninges, spinal fluid, and a portion of the spinal cord with its nerves

(320)   **2.**   List four classes of congenital anomalies that may occur in the neonate. Give one or more examples of each.

   a. _____

   b. _____

   c. _____

   d. _____

(321)   **3.**   List the two classifications of hydrocephalus and describe the features of each.

   a. _____

   _____

   b. _____

   _____

(322)   **4.**   List two possible complications of shunts for treatment of hydrocephalus.

   a. _____

   b. _____

(322-323) **5.**   Why is it essential to frequently change position if an infant has an enlarged head due to hydrocephalus but has not yet had a shunt?

   _____

   _____

(323-324) **6.**   List signs of the two primary complications that may occur after shunt placement for hydrocephalus.

   a.   Infection of the shunt _____

   _____

   b.   Increased intracranial pressure _____

   _____

(324)   **7.**   What is the current recommendation for all women related to prevention of neural tube defects such as meningomyelocele?

   _____

   _____

Student Name _____

(326-327) **8.** Describe nursing observations and care for the newborn with spina bifida in each of these areas.

    a.   Care of the sac before surgical repair _____

           _____

    b.   Extremities _____

           _____

    c.   Head _____

           _____

    d.   Bowel and bladder function _____

           _____

    e.   Latex allergy _____

           _____

(326) **9.** What are the positioning options the nurse may use for a child with a myelocele or meningo-myelocele before surgical repair?

           _____

           _____

(328-329) **10.** Describe postoperative nursing care for the child with a cleft lip and/or palate repair.

    a.   Preventing injury to the operative site _____

           _____

    b.   Positioning _____

           _____

    c.   Prevention of infection _____

           _____

    d.   Emotional care _____

           _____

    e.   Pain relief _____

           _____

(329)   **11.**   Describe three ways of treating clubfoot.

a.   _____

b.   _____

c.   _____

(329-330) **12.**   Describe nursing care of the child who has a cast on both legs.

_____

_____

_____

_____

(330-331) **13.**   List four signs of developmental hip dysplasia in the infant.

a.   _____

_____

b.   _____

_____

c.   _____

_____

d.   _____

_____

(332-334) **14.**   What procedure should the nurse use to turn a child in a body cast (spica)?

_____

_____

_____

_____

_____

_____

Student Name _____

(334-335) **15.** a. Explain how and when the nurse will screen a newborn for phenylketonuria (PKU).

_____

_____

_____

b. An infant's PKU screening is positive. What confirmation test is done for positive results on a screening test?

_____

(335-336) **16.** Describe the manifestations of the listed inborn errors of metabolism, how they are diagnosed, and their treatment.

a. Maple syrup urine disease _____

_____

_____

b. Galactosemia _____

_____

_____

(336-338) **17.** Describe physical and developmental characteristics that may be seen in a child with Down syndrome.

a. Facial features _____

_____

b. Hands and feet _____

_____

c. Musculoskeletal characteristics _____

_____

d. Internal abnormalities _____

_____

e. Physical and intellectual development _____

_____

(337-338) **18.** Parents of children born with Down syndrome have special needs. Give examples of how the nurse could help parents meet these needs.

    a.   Resistance to infection _____

        _____

    b.   Hypotonic muscles and loose joints_____

        _____

    c.   Constipation _____

        _____

    d.   Grieving _____

        _____

(338) **19.** Describe occurrences in the pathophysiology of erythroblastosis fetalis.

_____

_____

(338-339) **20.**   a.   What drug can prevent development of erythroblastosis fetalis and who (mother or infant) should receive it?

_____

_____

    b.   List five circumstances in which the drug is indicated.

       (1) _____

       (2) _____

       (3) _____

       (4) _____

       (5) _____

(340-343) **21.** Explain related nursing care in each of the following areas if an infant must receive photo-therapy in an incubator rather than with a fiberoptic pad or blanket.

    a.   Eye protection _____

        _____

Student Name_____

        b.   Protection of ovaries or testes _____

             _____

        c.   Potential dehydration_____

             _____

(343)   **22.** Intracranial hemorrhage around the time of birth is usually caused by

_____ or _____ .

(343)   **23.** List signs that should make the nurse suspect that a newborn has had an intracranial hemor-
            rhage.

        _____

        _____

        _____

        _____

(343)   **24.** What are two possible permanent effects of an intracranial hemorrhage?

        a.   _____

        b.   _____

(344)   **25.** a.   What causes the infants of some diabetic mothers to be larger than expected for their
                gestation?

            _____

            _____

        b.   What are other possible outcomes for the infant when the woman has diabetes during
                pregnancy?

            _____

            _____

        c.   What blood test should the nurse expect to perform when an infant is born to a
                diabetic mother? What is the normal level for a newborn?

            _____

            _____

CASE STUDIES

1. A newborn who has a meningomyelocele has paralysis of the legs and is dribbling urine and stool.
   a. Identify four nursing concerns for the nurse caring for the baby.
   b. What can the nurse tell the infant's parents about the dribbling of urine and oozing of stool as it relates to skin care and future control of these functions?
   c. How should the nurse involve the parents in the infant's care in the newborn nursery?
   d. What related problems should the nurse observe for in this infant? What signs should make the nurse suspect that the problems have developed?

2. Four-month-old Dianna is brought to the hospital by her mother because she had a seizure this morning. The admission physical exam shows an irritable, thin, lethargic child who the mother says has been vomiting the small amount of formula she would eat. Her height and weight measurements are below normal and her head circumference is slightly larger than normal. Dianna has not had any health care since her birth in a distant city. The admitting diagnosis is suspected hydrocephalus.
   a. Is Dianna exhibiting any signs of increased intracranial pressure? List observations that would support your conclusion.
   b. List diagnostic tests that may be done to confirm this diagnosis.
   c. What nursing measures should the nurse take to promote skin integrity?
   d. How should the nurse position Dianna during and after feedings?

APPLYING KNOWLEDGE

1. If you have a pediatric patient with Down syndrome, compare the development of gross and fine motor abilities of that child with those of a child of the same approximate age who does not have Down syndrome. Has the child with Down syndrome had any of the associated problems such as respiratory infections, ear infections, or heart defects?

2. While in the clinical area, care for a child who has Down syndrome.

3. Observe the repair of a cleft lip or cleft palate.

4. Care for an infant receiving phototherapy with a fiberoptic pad or blanket.

5. Give $Rh_o(D)$ immune globulin (RhoGAM).

Student Name _____

REVIEW QUESTIONS

(321) **1.** A sign that should make the nurse suspect hydrocephalus in the newborn is

1. inability to sleep between feedings.
2. a patch of hair on the lower back.
3. axillary temperature of 100° F (37.8° C)
4. an enlarged fontanel or cranial sutures.

(322) **2.** Expected treatment for hydrocephalus is

1. placement of a shunt.
2. incision and draining.
3. liquid oral diuretics.
4. intravenous analgesics.

(323) **3.** Vital sign changes when an infant has increased intracranial pressure include

1. increased blood pressure and pulse, hyperventilation.
2. decreased blood pressure, pulse, and respirations.
3. decreased blood pressure and respirations, increased pulse.
4. increased blood pressure, decreased pulse and respirations.

(326) **4.** Before surgical repair, the usual position of a newborn with a meningomyelocele is

1. side-lying with the head slightly below the level of the heart.
2. prone, maintaining abduction with a pad between the legs.
3. supine with the crib flat to stabilize blood pressure.
4. supine with the legs widely abducted and thighs flexed.

(328) **5.** Which of the following nursing measures is appropriate for a 2-week-old infant who has a new cleft lip repair?

1. position on the abdomen or side
2. place in a car seat after each feeding
3. provide a premature-sized pacifier
4. limit visitors to immediate family

(328) **6.** A priority of postoperative nursing care for a 9-month-old infant who has cleft palate repair is

1. referral to a parent support group.
2. adequate nutrition.
3. keeping an intravenous line open.
4. continuous sedation.

(329-330) **7.** Appropriate care related to a new plaster cast for correction of clubfoot in the newborn is to

1. keep the infant snugly wrapped until the cast is dry to prevent hypothermia.
2. sprinkle powder into the dry cast to reduce skin irritation at the edges of the cast.
3. position with the feet lower than the level of the heart until the cast is dry.
4. observe the toes for pallor, cyanosis, reduced capillary refill, or cold temperature.

(330-331) **8.** When checking range of motion on an infant, what sign should make the physician or nurse suspect developmental hip dysplasia?

1. reduced thigh abduction
2. full abduction and adduction
3. equal gluteal creases in the back
4. limited flexion of one knee

(331) 9. A 2-week-old infant will be fitted with a Pavlik harness as treatment for developmental hip dysplasia. The mother asks the nurse about the harness and how it will help her baby. To reinforce the physician's explanation, the nurse should teach the mother that

1. keeping the hip bone within the hip socket helps the socket to become deeper.
2. the infant cannot have surgery for the condition until he is at least 8 weeks old.
3. the longer leg gradually becomes shorter to equalize the leg lengths before walking.
4. time spent in a cast is reduced if the baby is treated with a harness for a few weeks.

(343) 10. The nurse should suspect intracranial hemorrhage in a newborn because

1. the fontanel is of normal size but depressed.
2. muscle tone has become poor since birth.
3. the infant seems to be hungry much of the time.
4. both pupils are small and react to light when checked.

(335) 11. The child with PKU must be on a diet that is

1. low in fatty acids to promote intellectual development.
2. high in soluble fiber to reduce constipation.
3. low in phenylalanine to limit buildup of the protein.
4. fluid-restricted to reduce the wastes delivered to the kidneys.

(335) 12. Early identification of galactosemia is required to prevent

1. depletion of specific amino acids.
2. liver damage, cataracts, and mental retardation.
3. protein deposits in the adrenal glands and kidneys.
4. limitation of normal growth in height.

(338) 13. Appropriate nursing care for parents immediately after the birth of a baby who unexpectedly has characteristics typical of Down syndrome should include

1. reassuring them that future babies are unlikely to have this problem.
2. keeping the infant in the nursery until a definitive diagnosis is made.
3. spending time with them so they can best verbalize their concerns.
4. teaching them about life-long nutritional care the baby will need.

(327) 14. Parent-infant bonding in an infant with a meningomyelocele prior to repair can be enhanced by

1. encouraging the parents to talk to and touch the baby.
2. having the parents change the baby's diaper.
3. encouraging the parents to hold the baby near their skin.
4. helping a parent give the baby an admission bath.

(328-329) 15. The mother of a 2-week-old infant who is going to have a cleft lip repair asks if she will be able to hold her baby after surgery. The nurse should reply

1. "The baby can be held when she no longer needs the restraints."
2. "The baby cannot be held but you can talk to her and stroke her."
3. "Holding your baby helps to keep her content."
4. "You should hold your baby only during feedings."

Student Name _____

(339) **16.** An Rh-negative woman who gives birth to an Rh-positive infant should receive Rh$_o$(D) immune globulin (RhoGAM) no later than _____ hours after birth.

   1. 4–8   2. 16
   3. 24–36   4. 72

(335) **17.** Expected advice for the woman with PKU who is considering pregnancy is to eat a daily diet that

   1. contains additional high-fiber foods.
   2. contains adequate dairy products.
   3. provides added amounts of leucine.
   4. has low quantities of phenylalanine.

(337-338) **18.** The infant with Down syndrome is at increased risk for developing

   1. urinary tract infections.
   2. respiratory infections.
   3. kidney infections.
   4. meningitis.

(344) **19.** What complication is more likely for an infant of a diabetic mother within the first few hours after birth?

   1. intracranial hemorrhage
   2. hyperactive reflexes
   3. excessive urination
   4. low blood glucose levels

(344) **20.** Why might an infant of a diabetic mother be small for gestational age (SGA)?

   1. The placenta did not receive adequate perfusion during pregnancy.
   2. The fetus had episodes of hypoglycemia when the mother took insulin.
   3. The fetal pancreas does not make insulin if the mother takes insulin.
   4. The mother's diabetes causes small areas of bleeding in the placenta.

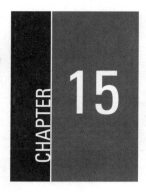

CHAPTER 15

Student Name _____

An Overview of Growth, Development, and Nutrition

Answer Key: Textbook page references are provided as a guide for answering these questions. A complete answer key was provided for your instructor.

LEARNING ACTIVITIES

1. Match the terms in the left column with their definitions on the right (a–f).

(349) _____ cephalocaudal

(349) _____ development

(349) _____ growth

(349) _____ maturation

(382) _____ parallel play

(349) _____ proximodistal

a. progressive increase in physical size
b. progressive increase in body function
c. total way a person grows and develops, dictated by inheritance
d. head-to-toe developmental pattern
e. central-to-peripheral developmental pattern
f. activity alongside another child or children

Answer as either true (T) or false (F).

(346) **2.** Children grow at a steady rate and in an orderly process. _____

(346) **3.** Fine and gross motor development proceeds from simple to complex. _____

(349) **4.** List the age range (in months or years) of each of the following stages.

    a. Fetus _____

    b. Newborn _____

    c. Infant _____

    d. Toddler _____

    e. Preschool child _____

   f. School-age child _____

   g. Adolescent _____

(349) **5.** Give a specific example of each type of developmental pattern.

   a. Cephalocaudal _____

   b. Proximodistal _____

(349) **6.** What are the two most rapid periods of growth after birth?

   a. _____

   b. _____

(349) **7.** Birth weight usually _____ by 6 months of age and

   _____ by 1 year.

(349-350) **8.** How does the percentage of body fluid change as the infant matures to adulthood? Why is it important for the nurse to know this?

   _____

   _____

   _____

   _____

(351) **9.** Why would a burn chart for calculating percentage of injured body surface area be inappropriate for a child with burns?

   _____

   _____

   _____

   _____

(350) **10.** Why are ear infections more common in young children?

   _____

   _____

   _____

   _____

Student Name _____

(352)   **11.** The Denver II assesses the _____ status of children from birth to 6 years of age in the following four categories:

a. _____

b. _____

c. _____

d. _____

Answer as either true (T) or false (F).

(352)   **12.** The Denver II is an intelligence test. _____

(352)   **13.** A low score on the Denver II indicates that a child has a developmental delay. _____

(352)   **14.** A *dysfunctional* family implies its members are not loving and caring. _____

(356)   **15.** List the components of the family APGAR.

A _____

P _____

G _____

A _____

R _____

16. Match the following behaviors with the correct stages of Piaget's theory of cognitive development (a–d).

(363)   _____ sensorimotor

(363)   _____ preoperational

(363)   _____ concrete operations

(363)   _____ formal operations

a. progresses from reflexes to intentional interaction with the environment
b. develops ability for hypothetical and abstract thought
c. views the world egocentrically
d. reasoning becomes more rational and systematic

(363, 367) **17.** How can parents' knowledge of growth and development help prevent accidents in children?

_____

_____

_____

_____

(367)   **18.** Why might a child who eats a vegetarian diet be anemic?

_____

_____

_____

_____

(371)   **19.** Children should continue on breast milk or iron-fortified formula until what age? _____

What is the earliest age that a child should begin whole milk? _____

(371, 374) **20.** Solids foods are introduced into the infant's diet at what age? _____

(374)   **21.** The first solid food introduced to infants is usually _____.

(371)   **22.** Why are restrictive diets not recommended for infants and young children?

_____

_____

(378)   **23.** One guideline for determining the appropriate amount of food to feed to children is

_____ tablespoon(s) of food for each year of age.

(378)   **24.** Primary dentition is completed by _____.

(379)   **25.** The first primary teeth erupt at _____ months.

Answer as either true (T) or false (F).

(380)   **26.** Carbohydrate consumption is the most important dietary consideration for dental health.

_____

(380)   **27.** The child should be encouraged to brush his or her teeth after eating sticky foods. _____

(379)   **28.** The American Academy of Pediatric Dentistry recommends that children have their first
dental visit by 1 year of age. _____

(380)   **29.** What are the causes of bottle-mouth caries? _____

_____

What is the prevention measure for them? _____

_____

Student Name_____

(381)   **30.**   What is the first-aid measure for traumatic loss of a permanent tooth?

_____

_____

_____

(382)   **31.**   What is the chief difference between the play of several toddlers (ages 1–2 years) and play of several preschoolers (ages 3–5 years)?

_____

_____

_____

THINKING CRITICALLY

1.   Observe a child in the clinical area. Based on the assessment, determine which of Erikson's stages of development the child is attempting to accomplish. Give at least three examples of observed behavior that support your choice.

2.   Using the information provided in Table 15-6 in the textbook and the Food Guide Pyramid (Figure 15-6), develop a meal plan for a 9-year-old child using foods unique to that child's ethnic background.

APPLYING KNOWLEDGE

1.   a.   Plot the height and weight of the following children on the growth chart (Figure 15-4 in the textbook).

Age	Height	Weight
2 years (boy)	33 in.	26 lb
4 years (girl)	38 in.	43 lb
8 years (boy)	52 in.	60 lb
12 years (girl)	58 in.	65 lb

b.   What percentile does each of the above children fall into?
c.   Which child would need further evaluation of his or her growth?

2.   Plan a menu for a 4-year-old hospitalized child on a general diet. Include in your plan serving size and how the food is best served.

3.   Perform a developmental assessment using the Denver II. Discuss your experience with your classmates.

REVIEW QUESTIONS

(349)   **1.**   A child must be able to sit before he can walk. This is an example of which directional pattern?

1. cephalocaudal
2. proportional
3. proximodistal
4. linear

(352)   **2.**   One of the most accurate indicators of biologic age is

1. height.
2. weight.
3. bone growth.
4. teeth eruption.

(363, 364)   **3.**   According to Piaget, the 7- to 11-year-old child is at which of the following stages of cognitive development?

1. sensorimotor
2. formal operations
3. concrete operations
4. proportional

(380)   **4.**   Dental caries are prevented through the administration of oral

1. iodine.   2.   fluoride.
3. sodium.   4.   iron.

(374)   **5.**   Most children are able to feed themselves using a spoon by age

1. 1 year.   2.   2 years.
3. 3 years.   4.   4 years.

(363)   **6.**   The theorist known for his work on moral development is

1. Freud.   2.   Kohlberg.
3. Sullivan.   4.   Piaget.

(355)   **7.**   A current comic strip depicts a family in which parents, children, and the children's grandfather live together. This is an example of a(n)

1. nuclear family.
2. alternate family.
3. extended family.
4. reconstituted family.

(373)   **8.**   Blood cholesterol levels below which level are considered acceptable in children and adolescents?

1. < 170 mg/dl
2. < 180 mg/dl
3. < 200 mg/dl
4. < 220 mg/dl

(378)   **9.**   Primary dentition is usually completed by

1. 18 months.
2. 2½ years.
3. 4 years
4. 6 years.

(349)   **10.**   An infant weighed 7 lb 15 oz at birth. What would the nurse expect this infant to weigh at 12 months of age?

1. 16 lb   2.   21 lb
3. 24 lb   4.   27 lb

(376)   **11.**   Which of the following statements would have the most positive outcome when counseling adolescents on nutrition?

1. "If you don't eat properly now, you may have heart trouble when you get older."
2. "You will get run down and sick if you don't eat properly."
3. "Shiny hair and good muscles are linked to good nutrition."
4. "If you eat nutritiously, you won't have acne."

Student Name _____

(382) **12.** Young children are playing with action figures in the hospital playroom. Closer observation reveals they are playing alongside one another, rather than interacting with each other. The nurse is observing

1. solitary play.
2. parallel play.
3. cooperative play.
4. creative play.

(380) **13.** A practice that should be discouraged is

1. allowing a 2-year-old child to brush his teeth.
2. feeding a 6-month-old infant iron-fortified cereal.
3. putting a 1-year-old infant to bed with a bottle of formula.
4. rocking a 9-month-old infant before bedtime.

(371, 374) **14.** Solids are generally introduced to children at age

1. 3 months. 2. 6 months.
3. 8 months. 4. 10 months.

(374) **15.** A parent asks when her 3-month-old infant can switch from iron-fortified formula to milk. The best nursing response is

1. "Switch to milk when you introduce solid foods."
2. "The baby can have milk when she can drink from a cup."
3. "Milk can be given at 6 months of age."
4. "Infants can drink milk after their first birthday."

(352) **16.** A 4-year-old child had a low score on the Denver II. The nurse understands that this finding indicates

1. the need for further evaluation.
2. the child has a cognitive impairment.
3. there is a problem with the child's speech.
4. the child has a developmental delay.

Student Name _____

The Infant

Answer Key: Textbook page references are provided as a guide for answering these questions. A complete answer key was provided for your instructor.

LEARNING ACTIVITIES

1. Match the terms in the left column with their definitions on the right (a–h).

(395) _____ colic

(393) _____ creeping

(398) _____ extrusion reflex

(386) _____ grasp reflex

(403) _____ object permanence

(386) _____ parachute reflex

(386, 392) _____ pincer grasp

(386) _____ prehension

a. closure of the hand when the palm is touched or stroked

b. thrusting tongue movements that automatically push food out of the mouth

c. extension of both arms when thrust downward in the prone position

d. ability to grasp objects between all fingers of one hand and the opposing thumb of the same hand

e. self-propelled forward movement carrying trunk above and parallel to floor

f. accurate and coordinated opposition of index finger and thumb of same hand

g. infant can remember that an object exists, even if it is out of sight

h. unexplained episodes of crying and irritability in an otherwise healthy infant

(386) **2.** How does sucking benefit a young infant?

a. _____

b. _____

(386) **3.** How can the nurse help meet the infant's sucking needs during the following?

a. Oral feedings _____

_____

_____

b.   Intravenous fluid therapy_____

_____

_____

(386)   **4.**   a.   The primary need for normal personality development during infancy is to acquire a

sense of _____.

b.   What can the nurse teach parents about meeting this need of their infant?

_____

_____

(387)   **5.**   Appropriate sensory stimulation is needed to promote what type of infant development?

a.   _____

b.   _____

(387-394)   **6.**   State the approximate age when the following events in an infant's growth and development are likely to occur.

a.   _____ months: briefly holds head erect and in the midline of body

b.   _____ months: can pull self up to standing

c.   _____ months: should have first DTP (diphtheria, tetanus, pertussis) inoculation

d.   _____ months: two lower central incisors; begins to crawl; transfers objects from one hand to the other

e.   _____ months: birth weight tripled; may walk

f.   _____ months: sits alone; pincer grasp

g.   _____ months: walks holding furniture; deliberately throws objects on floor

h.   _____ months: turns from back to side

i.   _____ months: can place a toy in small container

j.   _____ months: "jumps" when in lap of caregiver

Student Name_____

(397) **7.** Why should most infants not be placed in the prone position for sleep?

_____

_____

_____

_____

(398) **8.** What are three points that the nurse should emphasize to the parents to promote childhood immunization?

a. _____

b. _____

c. _____

(398) **9.** What guidance can the nurse give new parents who are concerned about whether their baby is receiving an adequate diet of breast milk or formula?

a. _____

b. _____

c. _____

(398) **10.** List four assessments that the health care provider may use to gauge the adequacy of an infant's nutrition.

a. _____

b. _____

c. _____

d. _____

(398) **11.** List health benefits for breastfeeding an infant.

a. _____

b. _____

c. _____

d. _____

(401)   **12.**   What food should be avoided for 2 years to prevent botulism in infants and young children?

_____

(399-400) **13.** a.   What is the current recommendation about when solid foods may be introduced to the infant's diet?

_____

_____

b.   Why is this age a good age to begin introducing solid foods?

_____

_____

(400)   **14.** a.   What is the first solid food usually introduced to the infant?

_____

b.   Why is this food good as an introductory solid food?

_____

(400)   **15.**   How should parents introduce new solid foods so that an infant's tolerance or intolerance of the food can be identified?

_____

_____

(400)   **16.**   List six foods that are usually delayed until the baby is 1 year old.

a.   _____

b.   _____

c.   _____

d.   _____

e.   _____

f.   _____

Student Name _____

(401)   **17.** The United States is becoming more obese, causing multiple health problems in the popula-
         tion. Is feeding an infant a low-fat diet one answer to the problem? Give a reason for your
         answer.

         _____

         _____

THINKING CRITICALLY

1. A mother is concerned because her 4-month-old baby does not seem to be developing as
    quickly as her sister's baby, who is about the same age. What should the nurse tell this
    mother about infant development?

2. When caring for an infant in the pediatric unit, talk with parents about their baby's personal-
    ity. Is their infant irritable, crying with handling or other stimulation, or calm when handled
    or meeting new people? How does the infant's behavior affect the parents or other family
    members?

3. Ask several parents how they cared for their colicky infant. How long did the infant have
    colic? How did it affect the family?

CASE STUDIES

1. You are answering questions from the parents of Sarah, a healthy newborn, in each of the
    following areas. Formulate appropriate parent teaching.
    a. Immunizations (first year) (In addition to your text, see the American Academy of
        Pediatrics web site at www.aap.org for the latest updates about immunization
        recommendations.)
    b. Sleeping all night
    c. Colic

2. Danny, 6 months old, is visiting the clinic for his immunizations and checkup. His parents
    will begin feeding "solid" foods now. What should you teach his parents in each of the
    following areas?
    a. Order of introducing solid foods
    b. Foods to avoid and how long to avoid them
    c. Avoiding infections acquired from foods

APPLYING KNOWLEDGE

1. Determine the most common infant formulas recommended by physicians or pediatric
    nurse-practitioners in your clinical facility. What special infant formulas are readily available
    in the newborn nursery or the pediatric unit and when are these prescribed? Check a gro-
    cery, drug, or discount store to compare prices for each formula.

REVIEW QUESTIONS

(386)   **1.** The priority need in personality development during the first year is to acquire

1. fear when meeting strangers.
2. mastering self-feeding.
3. trust in the primary caregivers.
4. consistency of sleeping, waking, and feeding.

(387-388) **2.** The primary use of growth and development guidelines is to

1. help parents anticipate their child's changing needs.
2. compare children of similar ages with each other.
3. predict general intelligence and school performance.
4. identify the child who is mentally retarded.

(393)   **3.** Which developmental milestone is expected for the child's age?

1. Passes a toy from one hand to the other at 3 months.
2. Uses the root reflex to seek the nipple at 5 months.
3. Sits steadily and without support at 6 months.
4. Pulls self to standing position at 10 months.

(386, 395) **4.** The mother of a 2-month-old is bringing her to the office for a routine checkup and immunizations. She says the baby cries quite a bit but she just lets her cry so she won't become "spoiled." As a nurse, the best response is to

1. tell the mother she should also lower the lights and play soft music or other "white noise."
2. explain that babies this young cannot be spoiled, then give her some ideas to help soothe the baby.
3. encourage the mother to continue helping her baby become more independent.
4. reassure the mother that she probably just has an irritable baby, but that this phase will not continue for long.

(397)   **5.** The best position for an infant to sleep in is

1. on the abdomen.
2. sitting in an infant seat.
3. on the parents' bed.
4. side-lying or supine.

(399)   **6.** If a parent wants to microwave formula before feeding, the nurse should

1. explain that microwaving overheats the formula because of its fat content and can cause severe burns.
2. tell the parent that cold formula preserves the nutrients better than heating it.
3. advise the parent to wait until the infant takes at least 8 ounces of formula at each feeding.
4. teach guidelines for microwaving and caution the parent to test the temperature of the formula before feeding.

Student Name _____

(388)   7.   The primary focus of regular infant health care is to

1. prevent disease.
2. accelerate development.
3. delay onset of allergies.
4. assess growth rate.

(402)   8.   A mother wants to know if she can keep leftover baby food in a jar. Choose the best nursing response.

1. "If you heard a definite 'pop' when opening the jar, refrigerating leftovers is safe."
2. "Refrigerate the leftover food within 2 hours after it is opened."
3. "When the baby has eaten all she wants from the jar, promptly refrigerate the remainder."
4. "Remove the amount of food you think the baby will eat from the jar and refrigerate the rest."

(398-399)   9.   A formula often prescribed for the infant who cannot tolerate cow's milk formulas is based on

1. goat's milk.
2. soy.
3. rice.
4. artificial protein.

(400)   10.   A nurse counsels a mother who is starting her baby on solid foods that she should wait _____ days before introducing the next food.

1. 1–2   2. 3
3. 4–7   4. 14

(389)   11.   Social development that is common for the 2-month-old infant is

1. responsive smiling.
2. laughing aloud.
3. recognizing his/her own name.
4. anxiety around strangers.

(400)   12.   When bringing her 9-month-old baby in for a checkup, a new mother asks if she can feed the baby puréed fish since this is a low-fat food that is a staple in the family's diet. The best response of the nurse is

1. "It is never too early to begin a heart-healthy diet."
2. "Fish protein is one of the best quality proteins available."
3. "You can try, but many infants dislike the taste of fish."
4. "Fish is more likely than other meats to cause allergies."

(392)   13.   The parents should make safety preparations prior to the time their infant crawls, usually about age

1. 4 months.   2. 7 months.
3. 9 months.   4. 12 months.

(399, 402)   14.   Which is the most important teaching about use of the microwave for heating infant food?

1. Use less time than would be needed for larger pieces of food.
2. Rotate the food two or more times while warming it.
3. Avoid heating foods that are higher in fat, such as meat.
4. Test the temperature of any warmed food on the inner wrist.

(400)   15.   A fruit that should be delayed until after the infant's first birthday is

1. strawberries.
2. applesauce.
3. apricots.
4. pears.

(403)   16.   Considering safety when choosing toys for a 5-month-old, one should assume that all of them will go into the baby's

1. tub.   2. food.
3. mouth.   4. bed.

(389)   **17.** Minor head lag when pulling a 1-month-old infant to the sitting position

1. is an expected finding.
2. demonstrates prematurity.
3. identifies poor nutrition.
4. suggests developmental delay.

(394)   **18.** A mother is concerned because her 1-year-old, who was 7 pounds (3178 g) at birth is "getting fat." The baby now weighs 21 pounds and all developmental milestones have been reached at appropriate ages. What should the nurse tell the mother about her baby's weight?

1. The weight at 12 months is about twice the birth weight.
2. The baby's weight gain is what is expected at this age.
3. A low-fat diet helps avoid being overweight later in life.
4. Infants normally weigh about 25 pounds by 1 year.

(395-397)   **19.** The nurse can reassure parents that their infant's colic will probably not last beyond the age of

1. 1 month.   2. 3 months.
3. 6 months.   4. 9 months.

(392)   **20.** The baby can usually be offered finger foods such as Zwieback crackers beginning at about age

1. 3 months.   2. 5 months.
3. 7 months.   4. 9 months.

(393)   **21.** A good initial method to deal with a 9-month-old infant who is attracted to a dangerous situation is to

1. shout a quick, loud "no."
2. take his favorite toys away.
3. spank him with one light blow.
4. distract him from the situation.

CHAPTER 17

Student Name _____

The Toddler

Answer Key: Textbook page references are provided as a guide for answering these questions. A complete answer key was provided for your instructor.

LEARNING ACTIVITIES

1. Match the terms in the left column with their definitions on the right (a–g).

   (411) _____ autonomy

   (420) _____ cooperative play

   (420) _____ egocentric

   (405) _____ negativism

   (420) _____ parallel play

   (405) _____ ritualism

   (409) _____ separation anxiety

   a. independent play in company of other children
   b. playing with other children
   c. consistent, recurring pattern of behavior
   d. independent functioning
   e. thinking in reference to oneself
   f. frequent reaction of "no"
   g. protest, despair, and detachment related to temporary absence of caregiver

(405-408) 2. What age is the toddler is expected to achieve each developmental milestone?

   a. Can undress self, throws ball _____

   b. All deciduous teeth are erupted; complete bowel and bladder control _____

   c. Imitates adults' activities, holds spoon _____

(405) 3. According to Erickson, the major developmental task for the toddler is to acquire

   _____ and overcome _____ and

   _____.

(408)   **4.**   What are the expected average vital signs for a 2-year-old?

    a.   Pulse: _____ to _____ bpm

    b.   Respirations: _____ to _____ breaths/minute

    c.   Blood pressure: _____ mm Hg

(412)   **5.**   What is a good guideline to teach parents about using "time out" with children?

_____

(411)   **6.**   List two self-consoling behaviors that toddlers exhibit.

    a.   _____

    b.   _____

(411)   **7.**   How should an adult talk to a toddler? Why?

_____

(413)   **8.**   List four indications of readiness for toilet training (in any order).

    a.   _____

    b.   _____

    c.   _____

    d.   _____

(414)   **9.**   Bladder training is more likely to succeed if the toddler stays dry for about _____ hours.

(414)   **10.**   Why is it important to teach the toddler generally recognized words to signal a need to use the bathroom?

_____

_____

_____

_____

(414)   **11.**   a.   What deficiency is more likely to occur if a toddler has excessive milk and too few solid foods?

_____

Student Name _____

     b.   This can result in what condition?

    _____

(414) **12.** Describe two characteristics of the toddler's eating habits.

     a.   Appetite _____

     b.   Food preferences _____

(415) **13.** What guideline can the nurse give parents about serving size of solid foods?

    _____

(412) **14.** List interventions that can assist parents with the toddler who resists bedtime.

     a.   _____

     b.   _____

     c.   _____

     d.   _____

     e.   _____

     f.   _____

(416) **15.** _____ are the leading cause of childhood death.

(416) **16.** List two methods that are mandated by law to prevent injuries in children.

     a.   _____

     b.   _____

CASE STUDY

    1. Tommy is a 2-year-old whose mother is frustrated because of his temper tantrums when he is disciplined. What can you teach Tommy's mother about discipline at his age? How can knowledge of normal growth and development be used to teach his mother about setting limits?

APPLYING KNOWLEDGE

    1. How can you help parents deal with the fears of their toddler? Why is it important for adults to control their own fears around a toddler? If you must do an unfamiliar procedure as a student (such as giving an injection) to a toddler, how can you control your own fears?

2. How can you use assessment of expected growth and development during the toddler years or other periods of childhood to provide better care when the child is hospitalized?

3. How can parents' knowledge of a child's expected growth and development help protect the child from injury? Give examples of advice you might give to parents of an 18-month-old child, a 24-month-old child, and a 36-month-old child.

4. How is full myelination of the spinal cord related to success of toilet training?

5. Use growth charts to determine if the physical growth of children you care for in clinical experience is normal.

6. Discuss daycare with classmates who are parents. Are they satisfied with the care their children receive? What, if any, problems have they had with daycare?

REVIEW QUESTIONS

(405, 408) 1. A first-time mother is concerned because she believes her 18-month-old son is not growing properly. Assessment indicates that the little boy's height and weight are average for his age. How can the nurse best advise her?

1. "He will soon resume the rapid growth of the first year."
2. "It is normal for a child's growth to slow down after the first year."
3. "Toddlers grow at inconsistent rates, much as adolescents grow."
4. "The physician will do testing if the child's growth remains slowed."

(411) 2. When helping a toddler choose clothing for the day, the best approach is to

1. ask him what he wants to wear.
2. ask which of two appropriate outfits he prefers.
3. select the best outfit for the weather.
4. remove all inappropriate clothing from his closet.

(411) 3. The position that best facilitates adult-child conversation is

1. at the child's eye level.
2. above the child's eye level.
3. standing while the child sits.
4. both seated at a small table.

(414-415) 4. When teaching parents of the toddler about eating, the nurse should stress that the toddler

1. prefers a variety of foods mixed on the plate.
2. must usually be coaxed to eat adequately.
3. eats one food for a while, then rejects it.
4. usually enjoys regular addition of new foods.

(412-414) 5. The mother of a 2-year-old asks the nurse whether she should begin toilet training now. The most appropriate nursing response is

1. "Your child is too young for toilet training to be successful."
2. "Does your child ever wake up dry in the morning?"
3. "Is it important to you and your family that the child be trained now?"
4. "It should be fairly easy to toilet train your child now."

Student Name _____

(416) **6.** Automobile child restraint devices should be used when the child

1. begins sitting in the rear seat.
2. crawls about in the car.
3. resists activity restraints.
4. travels anywhere in the car.

(417) **7.** Select the toy that is most likely to injure a toddler.

1. balloon 2. blocks
3. sand box 4. pull toy

(409-410) **8.** Which is the best description of a 2-year-old's speech and language ability?

1. Naming objects precedes the ability to describe what they do.
2. Some words such as swearing are used because they shock adults.
3. Talking to the child delays clear speech by limiting time to practice.
4. The child understands more than he or she is able to verbalize.

(405-408) **9.** Choose the best description of physical changes during the toddler years.

1. Head growth slows and chest growth continues.
2. Muscle size and strength remain steady.
3. Body temperature regulation is erratic.
4. Ability to fight infections is less than during infancy.

(416) **10.** The nurse can help reduce accidental injuries to toddlers by

1. providing toys that help accelerate motor development.
2. teaching parents about expected behavioral changes.
3. providing written information about common child hazards.
4. using restraints whenever the child is uncooperative.

(410) **11.** Select the assessment that should make a parent or health care provider suspect a communication disorder.

1. An 18-month-old child does not respond when his name is called.
2. A 15-month-old child can point to one picture when the parent calls its name.
3. A 3-year-old child can use plurals and pronouns correctly.
4. A 16-month-old child cannot use two-word phrases when appropriate.

(408) **12.** When assessing a 2-year-old child hospitalized for minor day surgery, the nurse should expect that the pulse rate will be about _____ bpm.

1. 60–80 2. 70-110
3. 125–135 4. 120–140

(412) **13.** When buying shoes for their toddler, parents should choose those that provide

1. a firm, straight sole to facilitate walking.
2. a strong arch to prevent "fallen" arches.
3. protection from objects that might injure the feet.
4. adequate movement of the heel within the shoe.

(416-419) **14.** Choose the recommendation that best helps to promote safety for the toddler.

1. Keep medicines on a shelf rather than on the countertop.
2. Provide stickers for each phone with the poison control center number.
3. Advise parents to have a cell phone with them when driving.
4. Do not use a hair dryer to dry the child's hair after shampooing.

(411, 412) **15.** A mother asks you what she should do about her 2-year-old child's temper tantrums. The best response is

1. "He is trying to tell you that he needs more attention from you and other important adults."
2. "If you let him get away with temper tantrums now, he will have more problems later."
3. "Have you tried rewarding his good behavior?"
4. "Try putting him in his room for about 30 minutes."

CHAPTER 18

Student Name _____

The Preschool Child

Answer Key: Textbook page references are provided as a guide for answering these questions. A complete answer key was provided for your instructor.

LEARNING ACTIVITIES

1. Match the terms in the left column with their definitions on the right (a–f).

(423) _____ animism

(423) _____ artificialism

(423) _____ centering

(431) _____ diurnal

(423) _____ egocentrism

(431) _____ enuresis

a. pertaining to daytime or waking hours
b. attributing lifelike qualities to inanimate objects
c. concentrating on a single aspect of an object
d. involuntary urination after the age at which bladder control should have been established
e. viewing everything in reference to oneself
f. belief that everything is created by people

(422-423) **2.** State the following typical vital signs in the preschool child.

a. Pulse: _____ to _____ beats/minute

b. Respirations: _____ breaths/minute

c. Blood pressure: _____ systolic and _____ diastolic

(427) **3.** Describe the following general characteristics of the 3-year-old child.

a. Sentences are _____ than at age 2 and they can express

_____ and ask _____.

b. They engage in both _____ and _____ play.

c.   May have a _____ attachment to the parent of the

opposite sex.

(427)   **4.**   A fear that is unique to this age group is a fear of _____.

(428)   **5.**   Describe the following general characteristics of the 4-year-old child.

a.   Prefers _____ toys.

b.   Plays with friends of the _____ sex.

(428)   **6.**   The 4-year-old child is _____ and likes to _____.

(428-429) **7.**   Describe the following general characteristics of the 5-year-old child.

a.   At age 5, children are more _____ and have more _____.

b.   Height increases by _____ inches and weight increases by

_____ pounds.

c.   May begin losing _____ teeth.

d.   Can play games that have _____.

(426)   **8.**   Masturbation in the preschool child is considered _____.

(429)   **9.**   Describe three ways children benefit from having limits set on their behavior.

a.   _____

b.   _____

c.   _____

(429)   **10.**   Effective discipline is designed to shift responsibility for control from the

_____ to the _____.

Student Name_____

(429)   **11.**   List three discipline methods that are often effective for the preschool child.

a.   _____

_____

b.   _____

_____

c.   _____

_____

(429)   **12.**   A time-out for a 3-year-old child should last _____ minutes.

(431)   **13.**   Thumb-sucking will not have a detrimental effect on a child's teeth if the habit is discontinued before _____.

(431)   **14.**   Describe the two types of enuresis.

a.   Primary _____

b.   Secondary_____

(431)   **15.**   List five possible causes of enuresis.

a.   _____

b.   _____

c.   _____

d.   _____

e.   _____

(434-435)   **16.**   The _____ age rather than the _____ age of the

child should be considered when selecting toys for the child.

(435)   **17.**   Hospitalization can be frightening to the preschool child because they are

_____. Their thinking is _____.

(435)   **18.**   Preschool children cannot fully understand cause and effect and they may perceive illness

and hospitalization as _____ for past behavior.

Answer as either true (T) or false (F).

(435)   **19.**   Hospitalized preschoolers may feel abandoned by their parents. _____

(436)   **20.**   It would be unusual for a preschooler to have enuresis during a hospitalization. _____

(436)   **21.**   Having the same nurses care for a hospitalized preschooler will lessen the stress of the experience for the child. _____

THINKING CRITICALLY

1.   What are appropriate ways to encourage a preschool child's desire to do things for himself while he is hospitalized in your clinical facility?

2.   How would you help parents who are concerned because their preschool child uses bad language?

CASE STUDY

1.   Sharon Giles is being discharged from the birth center with her second baby. Her 3-year-old son Shawn has visited with her and the baby for several hours since the baby's birth. Sharon expresses concern about Shawn's relationship with the new baby since he has previously been the only child in the home. What guidance should the nurse give Sharon about minimizing Shawn's jealousy during the first few weeks after she and the baby go home?

APPLYING KNOWLEDGE

1.   As you care for children in the clinical area, identify examples of egocentrism, animism, and artificialism in their behavior.

2.   Does your clinical facility have classes for siblings when a new baby is expected? What is included in the classes?

3.   What kinds of nursery schools are available in your area? Are there publicly supported nursery schools for children who are from low-income families?

4.   When you care for hospitalized children, are you able to use role modeling to teach parents? If you have not used role modeling, think of appropriate ways to use this parent teaching technique.

5.   If your clinical facility has a play therapist, observe this staff member's work with children.

Student Name_____

REVIEW QUESTIONS

(423) **1.** A preschool child falls off the swing and cries, "Bad swing! You made me fall!" This child's response is an example of

1. egocentrism.
2. intuition.
3. animism.
4. symbolism.

(423) **2.** Choose the best example of egocentric thinking.

1. "The airplane takes me to Grandma's."
2. "Water is blue because someone colored it."
3. "This big box is a truck."
4. "The moon sleeps during the daytime."

(427) **3.** Fears of preschool children are usually

1. similar to those of older children.
2. a result of the child's easy distraction.
3. less intense than when they were younger.
4. greater than those they had as toddlers.

(428) **4.** Favorite stories of preschool children are those that relate to their

1. aggressive tendencies.
2. self-centeredness.
3. daily experiences.
4. relationships with others.

(428) **5.** A healthy preschool girl asks her parents if she will die. The best response is to tell her that

1. people do not usually die until they are old.
2. she does not need to worry about dying.
3. parents usually die before their children.
4. she will not die for a long time.

(427) **6.** The best way for parents to handle masturbation is to

1. remove the child's hands from the genitals.
2. try to interest the child in another activity.
3. tell the child not to touch himself there.
4. ask the child why he is rubbing that area.

(429) **7.** One effective method of discipline for a preschool child is to

1. reward the child for good behavior.
2. give the child a light spanking.
3. review the reasons for discipline.
4. stop interacting with the child.

(430) **8.** Choose the most effective way for parents to deal with a preschool child's jealousy of her new brother.

1. Help her choose toys to share with the new baby.
2. Remind her of things she can do that the baby cannot.
3. Explain that she will soon love her new brother.
4. Ask her to share her room with the new baby at first.

(431) **9.** A child who sucks his thumb is unlikely to have damage to the mouth if the thumb sucking stops before

1. 3 years of age.
2. speech is established.
3. the first teeth erupt.
4. the permanent teeth erupt.

(431)   **10.** Choose the most appropriate teaching for parents of a child with enuresis.

1. Girls tend to have the problem because they have smaller bladders.
2. Most cases do not involve any abnormality and resolve without treatment.
3. Limiting the child's fluid intake to body requirements usually resolves the problem.
4. Most cases are the result of a minor urinary tract infection that is treatable.

(424)   **11.** According to Erikson, the developmental task of the preschool period is to achieve a sense of

1. trust.   2. autonomy.
3. initiative.   4. industry.

(423-424)   **12.** Delays or problems with language expression should be referred

1. before 5 years of age.
2. after completion of first grade.
3. to a psychiatrist.
4. only if the child has other delays.

(425)   **13.** Which type of play is imitative?

1. "Reads" from a story book that he or she has heard many times.
2. Says, "I'll be the mommy and you be the daddy."
3. Climbs up and down a jungle gym.
4. Participates in simple games with other children.

(428)   **14.** Choose the approximate age when children begin playing games that have simple rules.

1. 3 years   2. 4 years
3. 5 years   4. 6 years

(427)   **15.** Bedtime for the preschool child should include

1. flexibility in the time the child goes to bed.
2. a period of exercise after dinner.
3. warm milk.
4. a quiet activity such as a story.

(432)   **16.** A major cause of health problems in preschool children is

1. immunization reactions.
2. communicable diseases.
3. environmental allergies.
4. accidental injuries.

CHAPTER 19

The School-Age Child

Answer Key: Textbook page references are provided as a guide for answering these questions. A complete answer key was provided for your instructor.

LEARNING ACTIVITIES

1. Match the terms in the left column with their definitions on the right (a–d).

(438) _____ concrete operations

(440) _____ androgynous

(443) _____ latchkey child

(446) _____ preadolescent

a. period immediately preceding adolescence
b. sex role concept that incorporates both masculine and feminine qualities
c. logical thinking and an understanding of cause and effect
d. unsupervised children left at home after school

(438) **2.** The school-age child differs from the preschool child in that he or she is more interested in

_____ than in fantasy.

(438) **3.** According to Erikson, the school-age period is referred to as the stage of

_____.

(438) **4.** Concrete operations involve _____ thinking and an understanding

of _____.

(439) **5.** School-age children prefer friends of the _____ sex.

(439-440) **6.** Give approximate vital sign ranges for the school-age child.

a. Average weight gain: _____pounds per year

b. Average increase in height: _____ inches per year

      c.   Pulse: _____ to _____ bpm

      d.   Respiratory rate: _____ to _____ breaths/minute

      e.   Systolic blood pressure: _____ to _____ mm Hg

      f.   Diastolic blood pressure: _____ to _____ mm Hg

(440)   **7.**   How would the nurse advise parents to answer the school-age child's questions about sex?

           _____

(440)   **8.**   Describe information school-age children need in preparation for puberty.

      a.   Boys _____

           _____

      b.   Girls _____

           _____

Answer as either true (T) or false (F).

(443)   **9.**   Belonging to a group is important to school-age children. _____

(443)   **10.**   Latchkey children are at higher risk for accidents. _____

(444-445) **11.**   Describe the following typical characteristics of a 6-year-old child.

      a.   The attention span is _____.

      b.   Loss of _____ teeth occurs, along

           with eruption of _____.

      c.   Greater exposure to _____
           occurs with entry into school.

      d.   Requires _____ hours of sleep per night.

(445)   **12.**   The 7-year-old child prefers toys that are _____

           _____.

(445)   **13.**   Describe the following typical characteristics of an 8-year-old child.

      a.   Prefers friends of the _____.

Student Name _____

      b.   Enjoys _____ sports, but is

          a _____.

      c.   Secret clubs have strict _____.

(446)   **14.** Describe the following typical characteristics of a 9-year-old child.

      a.   _____ and _____

          _____ are common behaviors.

      b.   _____ sports are popular.

      c.   Needs _____ hours of sleep per night.

(446)   **15.** Describe the following typical characteristics of a 10-year-old preadolescent.

      a.   Strives for _____, but will take suggestions.

      b.   Ideas of the _____ are more important than those of the individual.

      c.   Takes greater interest in his or her _____.

(447)   **16.** Describe the following typical characteristics of 11- and 12-year-old preadolescents.

      a.   This period is one of complete _____.

      b.   The child has less ability to _____.

      c.   The child has _____ permanent teeth.

(451)   **17.** How would the nurse advise parents of a school-age child about homework?

      _____

Answer as either true (T) or false (F).

(451)   **18.** Children with an allergy to animal dander should not have a pet. _____

(451)   **19.** Children older than 7 years can be responsible for caring for a pet. _____

(451)   **20.** Having a pet can foster a sense of responsibility and encourage socialization for a shy child. _____

THINKING CRITICALLY

1.   For each category listed below, describe one or two ways the nurse can incorporate the needs of the school-age child into care during hospitalization.
     a.   Encouraging decision-making
     b.   Need for inclusion in a group

CASE STUDIES

1.   Rebecca, 6 years old, is receiving her booster immunizations before starting school. Her mother tells you that she is concerned about how Rebecca will adjust to school because it is the first time she will be away from home for a significant part of the day. How can you help her mother prepare Rebecca for school?

2.   Kyle, 10 years old, is hospitalized in skeletal traction with a badly fractured wrist and humerus that he suffered when playing street hockey with his friends. Kyle says he is really unhappy about being away from his friends during summer vacation. The boys spend most of the warm hours of the day at the public pool and either skate or ride their bikes until dark. What safety teaching does Kyle need? How can you use knowledge of preadolescent growth and development to teach Kyle and his family about safety? What can you do to meet his needs for companionship with his friends?

APPLYING KNOWLEDGE

1.   Observe how experienced nurses prepare children of different ages for medical procedures. Identify ways they use knowledge of growth and development when caring for children of different ages but with similar medical conditions.

2.   Watch television programs and evaluate them critically for positive and potentially harmful influences on children. Consider the following factors:
     a.   Stimulating the child's imagination
     b.   Materialistic focus
     c.   Stereotypes (gender, age, race, and family structure)
     d.   Violent content

Student Name_____

REVIEW QUESTIONS

(438) **1.** The school-age child who has few experiences of success is likely to develop a sense of

1. dependence.
2. inferiority.
3. trust.
4. industry.

(439) **2.** Which best describes physical growth of the school-age child?

1. Rapid growth occurs from 6–9 years of age, then slows.
2. Slow growth continues until just before puberty.
3. Height increases faster than weight.
4. Height and weight remain stable until the onset of puberty.

(440) **3.** Choose the normal characteristics of vital signs that the nurse should expect when assessing a 9-year-old girl.

1. Blood pressure and pulse are higher than those of boys the same age.
2. Blood pressure, pulse, and respirations are close to adult levels.
3. Blood pressure is higher, but pulse and respirations are lower than the adult.
4. Blood pressure, pulse, and respirations are higher than those of a 6-year-old girl.

(440) **4.** The best way to teach a child about sex is

1. before they ask any questions.
2. at their level of understanding.
3. as part of the school curriculum.
4. using terms used in the peer group.

(444) **5.** The most significant physical development at age 6 years is

1. loss of the primary teeth.
2. elongation of the face.
3. better infection resistance.
4. rapid growth in height.

(446) **6.** Worries and minor compulsions are more common at the age of

1. 6 years.   2. 7 years.
3. 9 years.   4. 11 years.

(447) **7.** A preadolescent is more likely to accept her parents' decision if

1. she understands why her parents made the decision.
2. the parents do not change decisions once they are made.
3. the parents carefully control the child's friends.
4. her friends have values similar to her own family's.

(442, 446) **8.** Choose the most appropriate safety teaching related to a 7-year-old child's use of a bicycle.

1. Use training wheels until balance is well-established.
2. Select a well-fitting helmet in the child's choice of color and design.
3. Restrict riding to light- or moderate-traffic streets near home.
4. Do not allow the child to ride with friends who might distract him or her.

(440) **9.** The preadolescent girl should have supplies for menstruation

1. before her first menstrual period.
2. as soon as she knows how heavy her flow is.
3. when her friends are prepared for theirs.
4. about six months after breast development begins.

(446)   **10.**   Which characteristic is typical of many 9-year-old children?

1.   Enjoy secret codes and rituals with friends.
2.   Start projects, but rarely complete them.
3.   Participate in intense teasing of the opposite sex.
4.   Argue and are bossy toward other children.

(443, 449)   **11.**   A group of 8- and 9-year-old boys has formed a "club." The boys have a secret password and handshake before they will meet. Parents should interpret this behavior as

1.   typical for children in this age group.
2.   a way to avoid being around adults.
3.   preceding criminal-type gang membership.
4.   rebellion against bossy older children.

(446)   **12.**   A father is concerned because his 9-year-old son has developed the habit of wrinkling his nose unconsciously. The nurse should tell the father that his son

1.   may have a nerve problem and should be seen by a physician.
2.   cannot get adequate adult attention without taking this action.
3.   is probably doing this because of unresolved tension.
4.   should be corrected any time he is caught doing this action.

(450)   **13.**   A school-age child has an adult "hero" of the same sex. What is the most appropriate interpretation of this behavior?

1.   The child feels insecure and inadequate around other children.
2.   Identifying with adults of the same sex is common at this time.
3.   Molestation or sexual abuse by the adult should be considered.
4.   The child is exploring various career and lifestyle options.

(445)   **14.**   Which statement characterizes the 8-year-old child?

1.   Eight-year-olds are totally disorganized.
2.   They are beginning to take an increased interest in their appearance.
3.   At this age, children are quieter and more modest than the year before.
4.   They like competitive sports, but are poor losers.

CHAPTER 20 The Adolescent

Answer Key: Textbook page references are provided as a guide for answering these questions. A complete answer key was provided for your instructor.

LEARNING ACTIVITIES

1. Match the terms in the left column with their definitions on the right (a–g).

(455) _____ adolescence

(456) _____ androgens

(456) _____ estrogens

(459) _____ menarche

(456) _____ puberty

(456) _____ growth spurt

(462) _____ self-concept

a. one's view of oneself
b. rapid period of growth in which a body reaches adult height and weight
c. first menstrual period
d. period during which reproductive organs become functional
e. female sex hormones
f. male sex hormones
g. period beginning with appearance of secondary sex characteristics and ending with physical and emotional maturity

(456) 2. In the formal operations stage of cognitive development, late adolescents are capable of

_____ reasoning.

(456) 3. One of the strongest needs of adolescents is _____.

(456) 4. Define *preadolescence*. _____

_____

(459) 5. Puberty occurs earlier in which gender? _____

(459) 6. The first change of puberty in a boy is _____

_____.

(459)   **7.**   Boys begin sperm production at about _____ years of age.

(459, 460) **8.**   Two important cancer detection tests that are appropriately taught during adolescence are

the _____ and

_____ self-examinations.

(459)   **9.**   A girl's first menstrual period is called _____.

(460)   **10.**   Erikson identifies the major task of adolescence as _____.

(460)   **11.**   _____ is
required for the adolescent to establish his or her own identity.

(462)   **12.**   Describe several possible adult outcomes if the adolescent does not achieve his or her own
identity.

_____

_____

_____

_____

Answer as either true (T) or false (F).

(463)   **13.**   Adolescents think everyone is looking at them. _____

(463)   **14.**   An adolescent's preoccupation with his or her appearance is a normal behavior. _____

(463-464) **15.**   How can cliques facilitate adolescent peer relationships? _____

_____

(465)   **16.**   State ways parents can help their teenager develop increased responsibility in each of the
following areas.

a.   Routine tasks _____

_____

_____

b.   Managing money _____

_____

Student Name_____

(468)   **17.**   List two factors that increase the risk for nutritional deficiencies during adolescence.

      a.   _____

           _____

      b.   _____

           _____

(468)   **18.**   An adolescent's diet is most likely to be deficient in which three nutrients?

      a.   _____

      b.   _____

      c.   _____

(470)   **19.**   The primary safety risk to the adolescent is related to use of a(n)_____.

(463)   **20.**   Psychosocial milestones that must be accomplished during adolescence include the five "I"s.

      a.   _____

      b.   _____

      c.   _____

      d.   _____

      e.   _____

(472)   **21.**   A change in school performance, appearance, and behavior can be a warning sign of

      _____.

THINKING CRITICALLY

    1.   A 15-year-old girl is at the pediatrician's office for a well-child examination. After you measure her weight, she tells you she is worried about being fat. Her weight is at the 75th percentile for her age. How would you respond to the girl's comment?

    2.   You are assigned to care for a 14-year-old boy. He responds to your questions with one-word answers. What strategies would you use to establish a rapport with this adolescent?

CASE STUDIES

1. John's mother is worried about the change for the worse in the behavior of her only child. "Our family has always enjoyed many activities together, but now John only wants to be with his friends. He doesn't seem to care that his clothes look bizarre, and yet he's constantly fussing with his hair. He never seems to pay attention. I'm afraid his grades will fall and he won't get into a good college." Can you help John's mother understand his behavior? What guidance might be appropriate for her?

2. Mary Lou, 15 years old, confides to you that she and her boyfriend have had sex a few times. Mary Lou is concerned about getting pregnant, but does not know much about contraception. She says that talking to her parents about sex and contraception is out of the question. How can you help Mary Lou make responsible decisions concerning her sexuality? What problems have you seen in adolescents who become parents?

APPLYING KNOWLEDGE

1. Observe a group of young adolescents. Identify behaviors in the group that demonstrate the following.
    a. Efforts to develop an identity
    b. Preoccupation with self
    c. Cultural variations

2. Obtain statistics for your state and city about the number of vehicle accidents in which teenagers were involved. If possible, determine how long the young drivers had been licensed.

3. Visit community groups that focus on reducing gang violence among teenagers. Determine the approximate ages of gang members and how they identify themselves to one another and to rival gangs.

4. Obtain local statistics for violent deaths among teenagers. How many of these are thought to be related to gangs?

REVIEW QUESTIONS

(456) 1. Younger adolescents often have an awkward appearance because

1. maturation occurs earlier than in previous generations.
2. body parts grow and mature at different rates.
3. growth and development slows during adolescence.
4. self-consciousness causes the adolescent to slump.

(462) 2. A person who does not establish an identity during adolescence is more likely to

1. conform to a peer group for a prolonged time.
2. seek close relationships with others.
3. become insensitive to the needs of others.
4. have an overly superior self-image.

Student Name _____

(465) **3.** A parent can best help an adolescent make a wise decision by

1. explaining what he or she would have done when he or she was a teenager.
2. reviewing problems with the decision after the teenager makes it.
3. serving as a role model by making the decision for the teenager.
4. respecting the teenager's decision, even if he or she makes a mistake.

(463) **4.** Younger adolescents tend to be egocentric because they are

1. certain that their parents are ignorant.
2. believe no-one is paying attention to them.
3. preoccupied with their physical development.
4. proud of their greater responsibilities.

(460) **5.** The adolescent's peer group helps him or her move away from

1. same-sex friendships.
2. values of his or her family.
3. individual responsibility.
4. dependence on his or her family.

(465) **6.** Daydreaming in the adolescent should be interpreted as a

1. normal occurrence.
2. sign of insecurity.
3. symptom of depression.
4. desire to ignore parents.

(468-469) **7.** An adolescent who adopts a strict vegetarian diet is at risk for a deficiency of

1. carbohydrates.
2. vitamin C.
3. protein.
4. fiber.

(470) **8.** Most accidents in adolescence occur when they

1. participate in contact sports.
2. handle guns or knives.
3. drive a car or other vehicle.
4. work at part-time jobs.

(460) **9.** Tanner stages describe the

1. sequence of physical maturation in the adolescent.
2. change from concrete thinking to abstract thinking.
3. hormonal changes that cause ovulation and menstruation.
4. development of a mature gender identity.

(455) **10.** The major psychosocial task of adolescence is to develop a sense of

1. sexual orientation.
2. concern for other people.
3. family unity.
4. identity as an individual.

(463) **11.** A woman is worried because her 14-year-old son seems to be constantly in the bathroom, shampooing and styling his hair. She worries that her son may be homosexual because he is so concerned about his appearance. Choose the best counseling for this mother.

1. Homosexual thoughts and experimentation are normal during the early teens.
2. Boys are usually more concerned about their athletic abilities than their appearance.
3. She should be more concerned about why he does not want to be with his friends.
4. Teens are preoccupied with their appearance because of dramatic body changes.

(468)   **12.** The most important consideration when teaching a teenager about a healthy diet is to

1.   include information about nourishing foods at fast-food restaurants.

2.   focus primarily on nutrients that are most often deficient in a teenage diet.

3.   teach the importance of an adequate diet to better health during adulthood.

4.   explain that dieting during adolescence can result in lifetime weight-control problems.

CHAPTER 21

The Child's Experience of Hospitalization

Answer Key: Textbook page references are provided as a guide for answering these questions. A complete answer key was provided for your instructor.

LEARNING ACTIVITIES

1. Match the terms in the left column with their definitions on the right (a–d).

(484) _____ clinical pathway

(491) _____ emancipated minor

(479) _____ regression

(483) _____ siblings

a. brothers and sisters
b. loss of an achieved level of functioning to a past level of behavior
c. interdisciplinary plan of care that displays progress of the treatment plan for a patient
d. adolescent younger than 18 years of age who is no longer under the parents' authority

(475-476) 2. List three advantages of outpatient surgery for the pediatric patient.

a. _____

b. _____

c. _____

(476-477) 3. A child's reaction to hospitalization depends on:

a. _____

b. _____

c. _____

d. _____

e. _____

f. _____

Answer as either true (T) or false (F).

(477)   **4.**   Every child reacts differently to the hospital experience. _____

(477)   **5.**   During hospitalization, a caring and compassionate nurse can take the place of a child's primary caregivers. _____

(476)   **6.**   Hospitalization can be a positive experience for children. _____

(477)   **7.**   The three major stressors for children of all ages during hospitalization are:

     a. _____

     b. _____

     c. _____

(477)   **8.**   Separation anxiety is most pronounced in the _____ stage.

     9.   Match the stage of separation anxiety with the behavior that corresponds with the stage.

(477)   _____ protest   a.   Child is sad and depressed.

(477)   _____ despair   b.   Child becomes interested in his or her surroundings.

(477)   _____ denial   c.   Child cries continuously for "mommy."

(478)   **10.**   List three nonpharmacologic methods of pain reduction.

     a. _____

     b. _____

     c. _____

(479)   **11.**   Administration of acetaminophen in quantities exceeding the recommended maximum daily dose can cause damage to the _____.

Answer as either true (T) or false (F).

(478)   **12.**   Infants and children respond to drugs differently than adults. _____

(479)   **13.**   Addiction occurs quickly in children receiving opioids for severe pain. _____

(479)   **14.**   Children 7 years of age and older can be taught to use patient-controlled analgesia. _____

(479)   **15.**   Administering analgesics on an as-needed schedule is the most effective way to relieve a child's pain. _____

Student Name_____

(479)   **16.**   The nurse must calculate all medication dosages to determine if they are safe to administer to the child. _____

(479)   **17.**   Define *conscious sedation*. _____

(479-480)   **18.**   What advice would the nurse give to a parent who is concerned that her hospitalized toddler was drinking from a cup and now only wants his bottle?

_____

(481)   **19.**   List three things the nurse can do to lesson anxiety for the parents of a hospitalized child.

     a.   _____

       _____

     b.   _____

       _____

     c.   _____

       _____

(483)   **20.**   List three ways the nurse can decrease siblings' anxiety when a brother or sister is hospitalized.

     a.   _____

       _____

     b.   _____

       _____

     c.   _____

       _____

(487)   **21.**   Give two methods of decreasing the stress of hospitalization for an infant.

     a.   _____

     b.   _____

(487-489)   **22.**   List three examples of transitional objects that can be brought to the hospital for a 15-month-old child.

     a.   _____

     b.   _____

     c.   _____

(489) **23.** What guidelines should the nurse follow for providing explanations about hospital experiences to young children?

a. _____

b. _____

c. _____

(489) **24.** Preschoolers are particularly fearful of _____.

(489) **25.** Explain how the nurse would prepare a preschool child for abdominal surgery.

_____

(489-490) **26.** List two ways the nurse can foster a sense of independence for the hospitalized school-age child.

a. _____

b. _____

(490) **27.** Following treatments, what should the nurse encourage the school-age child to do?

_____

(490) **28.** Illness in the young adolescent is seen mainly as a threat to _____

_____.

(491) **29.** What factors should the nurse take into consideration when assigning rooms or roommates for a hospitalized adolescent?

_____

(491) **30.** Preparation for discharge begins _____.

(492) **31.** What should be included in the documentation when a child is discharged from the hospital?

a. _____

b. _____

c. _____

d. _____

e. _____

Student Name _____

(491)   **32.** List four suggestions the nurse can give parents who are concerned about behavioral problems arising with their children after hospitalization.

a.   _____

_____

b.   _____

_____

c.   _____

_____

d.   _____

_____

THINKING CRITICALLY

1. Prepare a care plan for a hospitalized toddler. Address the psychosocial needs of the child
and parents. Include nursing diagnoses, goals, and interventions.

2. Do you think parents have the right to know if their children are being treated for a sexually
transmitted disease? Discuss this with your classmates.

CASE STUDY

1. Scott, 15 months old, is admitted to the hospital with a diagnosis of croup. Both of his
parents work and care for two older siblings.
a.   What factors will affect Scott's reaction to hospitalization?
b.   What information will you collect in a developmental history?
c.   How will you use this information to provide nursing care to this toddler?
d.   Scott's mother confides to the nurse that she feels that this hospitalization could have
been avoided if she would have taken Scott to the doctor sooner. How can you best
answer the mother?
e.   Following admission to the pediatric unit, Scott's parents leave to make arrangements
for their other children. Scott cries continuously for his mother. What is your
interpretation of this behavior?
f.   Scott's parents takG"Turns spending the night with Scott but are unable to be with him
during the day. What fears and behaviors might the parents show because of their
separation from Scott?
g.   Scott's 5-year-old sister asks you if her little brother is going to die like when her
grandfather was in the hospital. How should you respond to this question?

APPLYING KNOWLEDGE

1. Involve a school-age child in a board game. How effective was this strategy with establishing rapport and communication with the child?

2. While you are in the clinical area, assess a toddler who is alone for signs of separation anxiety. What stage of separation anxiety corresponds to the child's behaviors?

3. Take a hospitalized child to the playroom. Compare the child's behavior while in the playroom to behavior in the hospital room.

4. Discuss with your peers how you feel when parents do not come to visit their hospitalized child. What could be some reasons for their not visiting?

5. Determine the laws in your state governing the treatment of minors.

REVIEW QUESTIONS

(477) 1. Separation anxiety is most pronounced in which age group?

1 infants
2. toddlers
3. preschool children
4. adolescents

(487) 2. The mother of a hospitalized toddler could best explain when she will return by saying, "I will be back

1. in 3 hours."
2. after your nap."
3. before six o'clock."
4. before you know it."

(489) 3. In most instances, unpleasant treatments on children should take place in the

1. playroom.
2. emergency room.
3. patient's room.
4. treatment room.

(481, 487) 4. A child who is anxious about hospitalization will probably benefit most from

1. a visit from Bozo the clown.
2. having her favorite toy brought from home.
3. having her favorite foods served at lunch.
4. opening a new gift each day.

(489) 5. Children in which of the following age groups would most likely feel their illness is punishment for something they have done wrong?

1. toddler
2. preschool
3. school-age
4. adolescent

(489) 6. Anxiety over surgery can sometimes be decreased by

1. not telling the child that he or she is having surgery.
2. allowing the child to meet the surgeon.
3. visiting the surgical area preoperatively.
4. riding on the stretcher before surgery.

Student Name _____

(491) 7. Parental consent for minors is not always necessary for the treatment of

1. minor cuts and abrasions.
2. psychologic disorders.
3. communicable diseases.
4. sexually transmitted diseases.

(491) 8. The mother of 3-year-old Jason is concerned because he has returned to diapers since he has been hospitalized although he had been potty trained. What should the nurse say to the mother?

1. "This is very unusual and I'm sure it is temporary."
2. "Keep him in his training pants and don't give in to him."
3. "Regression is normal in a sick child."
4. "Perhaps he has some type of urinary infection."

(489) 9. The nurse's best approach to prepare a toddler for a painful procedure is to

1. be truthful if it will be painful.
2. avoid frightening him by not telling him it might hurt.
3. begin preparing early so that he can ask questions.
4. have his mother explain what will happen.

(490) 10. Hospitalized school-age children who act out should be

1. placed in a private room.
2. disciplined by having restrictions put in place.
3. provided with positive direction and consistency.
4. ignored because this is a normal reaction to hospitalization.

(487) 11. After performing a painful procedure on an infant, the nurse should

1. swaddle the infant.
2. feed the infant.
3. return the infant to the parent.
4. change the infant's diaper.

(489) 12. A common reaction of the preschooler to hospitalization is

1. anger.   2. depression.
3. guilt.   4. fear.

(489-490) 13. The hospitalized school-age child should be allowed to participate in his or her own care in order to

1. decrease fear of bodily injury.
2. increase self-esteem.
3. allow some control.
4. increase responsibility.

(489) 14. Because of distance, the family of a 6-year-old child cannot be at the hospital with her. The nurse suggests that the family

1. hire a private duty nurse.
2. bring in photographs and special toys.
3. not tell the child that they will not be visiting.
4. not call the child because it would be upsetting.

(489) 15. What is the best approach to decrease a preschooler's anxiety about having his blood pressure measured?

1. Take the blood pressure while the child is sleeping.
2. Ask the child's mother to take the blood pressure.
3. Demonstrate the procedure on a doll prior to performing it on the child.
4. Tell the child that big boys and girls do not cry when they have their blood pressure taken.

CHAPTER 22
Health Care Adaptations for the Child and Family

Answer Key: Textbook page references are provided as a guide for answering these questions. A complete answer key was provided for your instructor.

LEARNING ACTIVITIES

1. Match the acronyms in the left column with their definitions on the right (a–d).

(514) _____ O.D.   a. right eye
                        b. both eyes

(514) _____ O.S.   c. total parenteral nutrition or
                          hyperalimentation

(514) _____ O.U.   d. left eye

(518) _____ T.P.N.

(494) **2.** What is implied when a parent or guardian gives his or her written informed consent for a child to receive medical treatment?

_____

(494) **3.** A consent form must be signed by the _____, the

_____, and a

_____.

(494) **4.** The nurse acts as a _____ in ensuring proper consent

has been signed _____ a procedure and that the child is given an age-appropri-

ate explanation of the procedure.

(495)   **5.**   List six safety measures applicable to the hospitalized child.

a.   _____

_____

b.   _____

_____

c.   _____

_____

d.   _____

_____

e.   _____

_____

f.   _____

_____

(495-496) **6.**   Name four safety hazards to avoid when caring for a hospitalized child.

a.   _____

_____

b.   _____

_____

c.   _____

_____

d.   _____

_____

(496)   **7.**   Identify three factors the nurse must consider when selecting the method for transporting a child from the pediatric unit to the radiology department.

a.   _____

b.   _____

c.   _____

Student Name _____

(496)   **8.**   Name two procedures for which the nurse might use a mummy restraint for an infant.

     a.   _____

     b.   _____

Answer as either true (T) or false (F).

(497)   **9.**   Bradycardia is often the first sign of shock in infants and children. _____

(497)   **10.**   Hypotension is an early sign of shock in children. _____

(497)   **11.**   Bradycardia is considered a medical emergency in infants and young children. _____

(498)   **12.**   Medication dosages in children are determined by the child's weight. _____

(497)   **13.**   A _____ fontanel may indicate dehydration and a _____ fontanel may indicate increased intracranial pressure.

(499)   **14.**   Apical pulses are advised for children under age _____ years and should be counted for

     _____ seconds.

(499)   **15.**   The width of the blood pressure cuff should cover _____ of the upper arm.

(501)   **16.**   Fever is defined as a temperature over _____°F/_____°C.

(501)   **17.**   The main complication of fever in infants and young children is the development of

     _____.

(503)   **18.**   To accurately measure the temperature of a 4-year-old child using a tympanic thermometer,

     the nurse would gently pull the pinna _____.

(503)   **19.**   Describe the procedure for weighing an infant.

     _____

     _____

     _____

     _____

(505)   **20.**   Describe the procedure for collecting a urine specimen from an infant.

_____

_____

_____

_____

_____

(507)   **21.**   What is the purpose of a lumbar puncture?

_____

_____

(507)   **22.**   Explain how a nurse should position a child for a lumbar puncture.

_____

_____

_____

_____

_____

(507)   **23.**   What information should be recorded after a lumbar puncture?

_____

_____

_____

(508)   **24.**   _____ is the most important variable in predicting response to any drug therapy.

(508)   **25.**   Why are drugs metabolized more slowly by infants and young children?

_____

(510)   **26.**   What is the most common way to calculate a safe dosage when administering medications to children?

_____

_____

Student Name _____

(513) **27.** Describe the procedure for administering medication to an infant with an oral syringe.

_____

_____

_____

(514) **28.** Compare the procedure for administering ear drops to children under 3 years of age and children 3 years of age and older.

_____

_____

_____

_____

_____

(515) **29.** Which site would the nurse use to administer an intramuscular injection to an infant?

_____

Why is this the preferred site?

_____

(516) **30.** The maximum volume that can be injected in one site to infants is _____.

(517) **31.** _____, _____, and

_____ catheters are tiny, flexible rubber

tubes inserted into a vein in the chest to establish long-term intravenous therapy.

(518) **32.** How frequently does the nurse assess a child's intravenous infusion? _____

(518) **33.** When intravenous fluids are infusing, the nurse observes the child's IV site for:

a. _____

b. _____

c. _____

d. _____

e. _____

(518)   **34.** Total parenteral nutrition is given to children who _____

_____.

(519, 524) **35.** Describe the procedure for giving a gastrostomy tube feeding.

_____

_____

_____

_____

_____

(523)   **36.** Describe the procedure for suctioning a child with a tracheostomy.

_____

_____

_____

_____

_____

(525)   **37.** Describe the care of the tracheal stoma and the changing of the tape around the child's neck.

_____

_____

_____

_____

_____

(525)   **38.** List five signs that might indicate a problem in a tracheostomy patient.

a. _____

b. _____

c. _____

d. _____

e. _____

Student Name_____

(525)   **39.**   What emergency equipment should be kept at the bedside of a tracheotomy patient?

_____

(525)   **40.**   What should be included in the documentation when assessing a child with a tracheotomy?

a.   _____

b.   _____

c.   _____

d.   _____

e.   _____

(528)   **41.**   What is the Heimlich maneuver?

_____

(528)   **42.**   How is the Heimlich maneuver performed on an unconscious child who is lying down?

_____

(528)   **43.**   Prior to surgery, infants should not be maintained on NPO status longer than _____

to _____ hours because of the risk of _____.

THINKING CRITICALLY

1.   You are assisting a registered nurse who is going to start intravenous fluids on a 3-month-old infant. The mother is crying and is not sure if she wants to be with the infant or to remain outside the room during the procedure. How could you support this mother?

APPLYING KNOWLEDGE

1.   Where would the following items and areas be found in the clinical setting?

a.   blood pressure machine
b.   diapers
c.   emergency cart
d.   intake and output sheet
e.   IV soluset
f.   oral medication syringe

g.   playroom
h.   procedure manual
i.   scales
j.   thermometer
k.   treatment room
l.   urine collection bag

2.   Assist a registered nurse when she starts an IV on a child.

3.   Care for a child with a tracheotomy tube.

4.   Care for a child receiving gastrostomy tube feedings.

5.   Care for a child with an IV infusing.

REVIEW QUESTIONS

(499)   **1.**   Pulse and respiration rates of children are

1.   lower than adults.
2.   the same as adults.
3.   higher than adults.
4.   lower at birth, but higher by age 3 years.

(513)   **2.**   Unpleasant-tasting medications can be mixed in

1.   orange juice.
2.   milk.
3.   jelly.
4.   cereal.

(513)   **3.**   An infant's diaper weighs 30 g. How many milliliters would you record on the intake and output sheet?

1.   15   2.   30
3.   60   4.   45

(523)   **4.**   When caring for a tracheotomy patient, the nurse should

1.   limit suctioning to no more than 15 seconds.
1.   apply suction as the catheter is being inserted.
2.   use a suction catheter that is approximately the same diameter as the tracheotomy tube.
4.   replace the suction catheter and water used to clear the catheter at the end of the shift.

(511)   **5.**   A child weighing 35½ pounds has a medication order for phenytoin PO at 8:00 AM. The recommended pediatric dosage is 3–5 mg/kg/day. A safe dosage for this child would be

1.   75 mg.   2.   105 mg.
3.   150 mg.   4.   200 mg.

(503)   **6.**   An infant should be weighed

1.   completely naked.
2.   with a diaper in place.
3.   wrapped in a receiving blanket.
4.   completely dressed.

(527)   **7.**   The neonate exposed to prolonged high oxygen concentrations is at risk for damage to the

1.   heart.   2.   eyes.
3.   brain.   4.   kidneys.

(499)   **8.**   Both the pulse and respirations of children should be counted for _____ seconds.

1.   15   2.   30
3.   45   4.   60

(499)   **9.**   The blood pressure cuff on a child's upper arm should cover

1.   one half of the upper arm.
2.   one third of the upper arm.
3.   two thirds of the upper arm.
4.   the entire upper arm.

Student Name _____

(514) **10.** A child has a medication order for Garamycin 2 drops O.D. twice daily. The nurse would administer the medication to the

1. right eye.   2. right ear.
3. left eye.   4. left ear.

(515) **11.** The preferred intramuscular injection site for infants is the

1. deltoid.
2. ventrogluteal.
3. vastus lateralis.
4. dorsogluteal.

(516) **12.** The maximum volume that can be given by intramuscular injection at one site to older infants and small children is

1. 0.1 ml.   2. 0.5 ml.
3. 1.0 ml.   4. 1.5 ml.

(518) **13.** Nursing assessment and documentation of the child receiving IV fluids should occur

1. every 15 minutes.
2. every 30 minutes.
3. hourly.
4. every 4 hours.

(524) **14.** After receiving a gastrostomy tube feeding, an infant should be placed in what position when returned to bed?

1. left side   2. supine
3. right side   4. prone

CHAPTER 23

Student Name _____

The Child with a Sensory or Neurological Condition

Answer Key: Textbook page references are provided as a guide for answering these questions. A complete answer key was provided for your instructor.

LEARNING ACTIVITIES

1. Match the terms in the left column with their definitions on the right (a–j).

(540)	_____ hyperopia	a. presence of blood in the anterior chamber of the eye
(541)	_____ hyphema	b. farsighted
(536)	_____ myringotomy	c. incision of the tympanic membrane
		d. involuntary movement of the eye
(548)	_____ nystagmus	e. adduction of arms, flexed on chest with wrists flexed, hands fisted, and lower extremities extended and adducted
(534)	_____ otoscope	f. edema and inflammation of the optic nerve
(548)	_____ papilledema	g. temporary disturbance of the brain followed by a period of unconsciousness
(540)	_____ strabismus	h. instrument used to view the ear
		i. rigid extension and pronation of the arms and legs
(559)	_____ concussion	j. cross-eyed
(560)	_____ decerebrate	
(560)	_____ decorticate	

(535) 2. An acute infection of the external ear canal is called _____

or _____.

Answer as either true (T) or false (F).

(535) 3. When a child has otitis externa, the tympanic membrane is erythematous. _____

(535) 4. Prolonged exposure to moisture is a precipitating factor of otitis externa. _____

(535) 5. Otitis media frequently occurs after a child has an upper respiratory infection. _____

(536) **6.** Explain why infants are more prone to ear infections than older children.

_____

_____

_____

(536) **7.** List the main symptoms of otitis media.

_____

_____

(536) **8.** List two possible complications of recurrent episodes of otitis media.

a. _____

b. _____

(536) **9.** Describe the treatment of otitis media.

_____

_____

(536) **10.** What teaching should be done when antibiotics are prescribed for children?

_____

_____

_____

(537) **11.** Complete bilateral deafness is usually discovered during _____, but

partial deafness may be unrecognized until _____.

(537) **12.** List some common signs seen in infants and school-age children that might indicate a hearing problem.

Infants

a. _____

b. _____

School-age children

a. _____

b. _____

Student Name_____

(538) **13.** List three strategies the nurse can use when caring for a hospitalized school-age child who is deaf.

      a. _____

      b. _____

      c. _____

(538) **14.** Identify one strategy to relieve a child's discomfort resulting from a change in altitude or barometric pressure during airplane descent.

_____

_____

(539) **15.** During a visual assessment, the nurse should observe the eyes for:

      a. _____

      b. _____

(539) **16.** Visual acuity can be tested by _____ to _____ years of age.

(539) **17.** Explain the goal of treatment of amblyopia.

_____

_____

_____

_____

_____

(540) **18.** Why might a child be embarrassed when being treated for amblyopia?

_____

_____

_____

(540) **19.** Untreated strabismus can result in _____.

(541) **20.** Describe the procedure for wiping secretions from the eye in the child with conjunctivitis.

_____

_____

(542)   **21.** How would the nurse position a child who has a hyphema?

_____

(542)   **22.** List the clinical manifestations of retinoblastoma.

_____

(542)   **23.** Neural tube development occurs about the _____ to

_____ week of fetal life.

(542)   **24.** What medication, when used during a viral illness, has been linked to Reye's syndrome?

_____

(545-546) **25.** Immunization against _____ is recommended for all children

between _____ and _____ to prevent sepsis.

(546)   **26.** List five signs and symptoms of meningitis.

a. _____

b. _____

c. _____

d. _____

e. _____

(547)   **27.** Nursing measures for the child with meningitis include:

a. _____

b. _____

c. _____

d. _____

(547)   **28.** List two measures the nurse should take to decrease stimuli when caring for a child with meningitis.

a. _____

b. _____

Student Name_____

(560) **29.** Identify the following illustrations as decorticate posturing or decerebrate posturing.

a. _____

b. _____

a.

b.

(548) **30.** The majority of brain tumors in children are located in the _____

_____.

(548) **31.** The manifestations of a brain tumor are directly related to the _____

and _____ of the tumor.

(548) **32.** Most brain tumors create increased _____,

producing symptoms such as _____,

_____, _____, and

_____.

(548) **33.** Preoperative care of a child with a brain tumor should address what body image issue?

_____

(549) **34.** Febrile seizures occur in response to a _____.

(549)   **35.**   What information should the nurse observe and record after a seizure?

a.   _____

b.   _____

c.   _____

d.   _____

e.   _____

f.   _____

g.   _____

36.   Match each classification of seizure with its description (a–d).

(550)   _____ generalized tonic-clonic   a.   temporary loss of awareness
seizure   b.   can be manifested by motor activities, sensory
signs, or psychomotor activity
(550)   _____ absence seizure   c.   repetitive muscle contractions
d.   has three phases: aura, seizure, and postictal
(550)   _____ partial seizure   period

(550)   _____ myoclonic seizure

(553)   **37.**   What is the term meaning a series of convulsions rapidly following one another?

_____

(553)   **38.**   The most common cause of status epilepticus is _____ .

(554)   **39.**   List four common causes of cerebral palsy.

a.   _____

b.   _____

c.   _____

d.   _____

(554-555) **40.**   List three clinical manifestations that might indicate a child has cerebral palsy.

a.   _____

b.   _____

c.   _____

Student Name_____

(558) **41.** List two approaches that parents of mentally retarded children can take to enhance their child's abilities.

    a. _____

    b. _____

(560) **42.** Four components of a neurologic check are:

    a. _____

    b. _____

    c. _____

    d. _____

(562) **43.** List three questions you might ask a 4-year-old child to help determine his or her level of consciousness.

    a. _____

    b. _____

    c. _____

(562-563) **44.** Name three things you could observe to test the motor ability of a child with a head injury.

    a. _____

    b. _____

    c. _____

(563) **45.** What special observations should be made of an infant with a head injury?

    a. _____

    b. _____

    c. _____

THINKING CRITICALLY

  1. You are assigned to care for a 5-year-old child who has a seizure disorder. When you walk into her room, she is watching TV. You are asking the child some questions when her body stiffens. She is unresponsive. Thirty seconds later, her arms and legs begin contracting and relaxing. What type of seizure is this child experiencing? What should you do at this time?

CASE STUDIES

1. Kevin, age 6 months, is admitted to the hospital with meningitis. He is placed in isolation, an IV is started, and he is on seizure precautions.
   a. How would Kevin be positioned for a lumbar puncture?
   b. What changes in Kevin's spinal fluid would confirm a diagnosis of meningitis?
   c. Kevin's temperature is 102.4° F. For what other signs and symptoms would the nurse assess?
   d. State at least 6 nursing interventions for Kevin.

2. Two-year-old Andrew has chronic otitis media with effusion. Audiometric testing shows a mild hearing loss. He is scheduled for a myringotomy with insertion of tympanoplasty tubes.
   a. How will this surgery improve Andrew's hearing?
   b. What should Andrew's parents know about care of a child with tympanoplasty tubes inserted?

APPLYING KNOWLEDGE

1. While in the clinical area, care for a child who is on seizure precautions. What are some of the special procedures you followed?

2. Observe the following in children in the clinical area.
   a. reflexes of a newborn
   b. gait
   c. finger–nose test

3. Care for a child with meningitis. Observe for neurologic involvement.

4. Assist with vision screening in your local school district.

5. Visit your local Easter Seal Society and observe the therapy of children with cerebral palsy. Find out what resources are available for these children.

REVIEW QUESTIONS

(536) 1. Children with tympanostomy tubes should
   1. be given antibiotics.
   2. avoid getting water in their ears.
   3. sleep on their backs.
   4. take a decongestant.

(539) 2. Visual acuity can be checked by age
   1. 2½–3 years. 2. 3–4 years.
   3. 4–5 years. 4. 5–6 years.

(542) 3. Early signs of Reye's syndrome include
   1. diarrhea and headache.
   2. vomiting and lethargy.
   3. nausea and malaise.
   4. hyperactivity and vomiting.

Student Name_____

(547) **4.** When taking the history of a child with encephalitis, it is important to note recent

1. cat scratches.
2. tick bites.
3. respiratory infection.
4. drug therapy.

(554) **5.** Cerebral palsy is

1. a form of mental retardation that does not improve with treatment.
2. a nonprogressive disorder that affects the motor centers of the brain.
3. always caused by a birth injury occurring in early gestational births.
4. related to lack of early childhood stimulation and is irreversible.

(546) **6.** The most common causative agent of bacterial meningitis is

1. *Haemophilus influenzae.*
2. *Streptococcus pneumoniae.*
3. *Neisseria meningitides.*
4. *Escherichia coli.*

(546) **7.** Which of the following are signs and symptoms of meningitis?

1. diarrhea and stiff neck
2. hyperactivity and vomiting
3. irritability and fever
4. loss of vision and nausea

(549) **8.** A 7-month-old child had a febrile seizure. Which statement would the nurse give to the infant's parents? "Febrile seizures

1. rarely occur before an infant's first birthday."
2. indicate an underlying neurological problem."
3. are usually controlled with phenobarbital."
4. rarely develop into epilepsy."

(563) **9.** Fluids are monitored in children with a head injury in order to

1. prevent renal damage.
2. control cerebral edema.
3. prevent aspiration.
4. decrease headaches.

(550) **10.** Nursing care for a child experiencing a seizure would include

1. attempting to hold the tongue.
2. administration of oxygen.
3. restraint.
4. turning on his or her side.

(552) **11.** A common side effect of Dilantin is

1. drowsiness.
2. gum overgrowth.
3. hyperactivity.
4. headache.

(538) **12.** When caring for a hospitalized child who is deaf, the nurse should

1. speak in a loud, clear tone.
2. stand close to the child and speak slowly.
3. speak at eye level with the child.
4. speak in an exaggerated tone.

(546) **13.** An infant brought to the emergency room with a high fever, irritability, and a high-pitched cry would immediately be evaluated for

1. retinoblastoma.
2. Reye's syndrome.
3. neuroblastoma.
4. meningitis.

(547) **14.** An appropriate nursing intervention for an infant with bacterial meningitis is

1. restrain the infant when awake.
2. position the infant on the right side.
3. keep the room quiet and indirectly lit.
4. place in isolation until discharged.

(563)   **15.** A child has a Glasgow coma scale score of 15. The nurse should

    1. tell the charge nurse immediately.
    2. change the position of the child.
    3. chart the results of the assessment.
    4. stimulate the child.

(562)   **16.** Parents of a child with a head injury should be advised to call their primary caregiver if the child

    1. falls asleep.
    2. develops a bump.
    3. vomits one time.
    4. cannot be aroused.

CROSSWORD PUZZLE

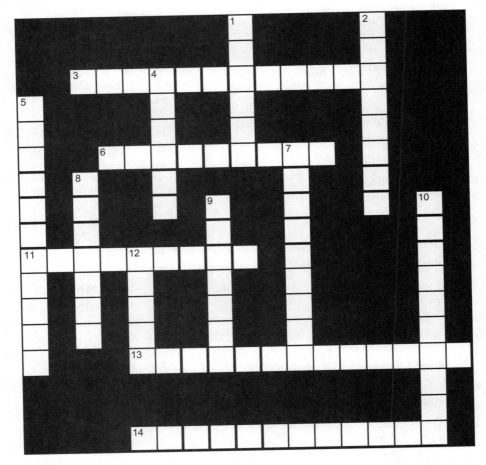

Across

(546)   **3.**   Involuntary arching of the back due to muscle contraction

(549)   **6.**   A short period of sleep following a seizure

(554)   **11.** Involuntary, purposeless movements

(554)   **13.** A group of nonprogressive disorders that affects the motor centers of the brain

(542)   **14.** Inflammation of the brain

Down

(549)   **1.**   A movement characterized by an alternating contraction and relaxation of muscles

(540)   **2.**   A reading disability that involves a defect in the cortex of the brain that processes graphic symbols

(545)   **4.**   Systemic response caused by bacteria in the bloodstream

(542)   **5.**   Removal of the eye as the standard treatment for retinoblastoma

(540)   **7.**   A reduction in or loss of vision in a child who strongly favors one eye

(541)   **8.**   The presence of blood in the anterior chamber of the eye

(549)   **9.**   Sudden, intermittent episodes of altered consciousness, lasting seconds to minutes

(540)   **10.** A condition where there is a lack of coordination between the eye muscles that direct movement of the eye

(549)   **12.** A movement characterized by muscle contraction

CHAPTER 24

The Child with a Musculoskeletal Condition

Answer Key: Textbook page references are provided as a guide for answering these questions. A complete answer key was provided for your instructor.

LEARNING ACTIVITIES

1. Match the terms in the left column with their definitions on the right (a–h).

(569)	_____ arthroscope	a. limited neck motion due to shortening of the sternocleidomastoid muscle
(568)	_____ genu varum	b. bow-legged or knees turned outward
(578)	_____ osteomyelitis	c. knock-kneed or knees turned inward
(569)	_____ contusion	d. tearing of subcutaneous tissue that results in hemorrhage, edema, and pain
(570)	_____ strain	e. a microscopic tear to a muscle or tendon
(568)	_____ genu valgum	f. infection of the bone
(579)	_____ osteosarcoma	g. bone tumor
(581)	_____ torticollis	h. endoscope for examining interior of a joint

(568) 2. Assessment of the musculoskeletal system in children who can walk includes:

a. _____

b. _____

c. _____

d. _____

(568) 3. It is normal for toddlers to have a _____ gait.

(569) 4. How would the nurse test the strength of a child's extremities?

_____

Answer as either true (T) or false (F).

(568)   **5.**   A newborn's feet may turn inward or outward. _____

(568)   **6.**   Children who do not walk independently by 12 months of age should be evaluated for a musculoskeletal problem. _____

(568)   **7.**   Young children may appear "bow-legged" until 5 years of age. _____

(569)   **8.**   A neurological assessment is part of a comprehensive musculoskeletal assessment. _____

(570-571) **9.**   List three types of traction used for children.

    a.   _____

    b.   _____

    c.   _____

(569)   **10.**   Identify three differences in the skeletal system of a child as compared to an adult.

    a.   _____

    b.   _____

    c.   _____

(569)   **11.**   The major signs of a muscle sprain are _____,

_____, and _____.

(570)   **12.**   Describe the treatment of a soft tissue injury.

_____

_____

_____

_____

13.   Match the types of fractures in the left column with their definitions on the right (a–d).

(570)   _____ simple

(570)   _____ compound

(570)   _____ complete

(570)   _____ greenstick

    a.   bone is entirely broken across
    b.   bone is broken but the skin over the area is not broken
    c.   open fracture in which the wound in the skin leads to the broken bone
    d.   incomplete fracture

Student Name _____

(570)   **14.**   Bryant's traction is used for treating fractures of the femur in children under _____ years

of age or under _____ to _____ pounds.

(572)   **15.**   You are performing a neurovascular assessment on a young child in Bryant's traction. Name three findings on the neurovascular assessment that should be reported immediately to the nurse in charge.

       a.   _____

       b.   _____

       c.   _____

(572)   **16.**   What is Volkmann's ischemia? _____

_____

_____

(573)   **17.**   A priority nursing responsibility in the care of a child with a cast or in traction is

_____.

(573)   **18.**   A neurovascular assessment of the toes of a child with a fracture who has a cast or Ace bandage includes checking for:

       a.   _____

       b.   _____

       c.   _____

       d.   _____

       e.   _____

       f.   _____

(573)   **19.**   Pain at the trauma site that is not relieved by analgesics may be a sign of

_____.

(571)   **20.**   Explain Russell's traction.

_____

_____

_____

_____

_____

_____

(571)   **21.**   Complete the following traction-related statements.

    a.   Weights are hanging _____.

    b.   Weights are out of reach of _____.

    c.   Ropes are on the _____.

    d.   Knots are not resting against _____.

    e.   Bed linens are not on _____.

    f.   _____ is in place.

    g.   Apparatus does not touch the _____ of the _____.

(578-579)   **22.**   Based on the signs and symptoms and treatment of osteomyelitis, list three appropriate nursing diagnoses for this disease.

    a.   _____

    _____

    b.   _____

    _____

    c.   _____

    _____

(579)   **23.**   The most common type of muscular dystrophy is _____

_____.

Student Name _____

(579) **24.** List three signs that might indicate a child has muscular dystrophy.

a. _____

b. _____

c. _____

(579) **25.** List two clinical manifestations of Legg-Calvé-Perthes disease.

a. _____

b. _____

(579) **26.** What would you tell the parents about the prognosis of Legg-Calvé-Perthes disease in their child?

_____

_____

_____

_____

(580) **27.** A diagnosis of osteosarcoma is confirmed through a _____.

(581) **28.** What are the goals of care of juvenile rheumatoid arthritis?

a. _____

b. _____

c. _____

d. _____

e. _____

(582) **29.** The two types of scoliosis are _____ and

_____.

(582) **30.** The Milwaukee brace must be worn _____ hours a day.

(583) **31.** Screening for scoliosis should be done before _____.

(583)   **32.** What does a screening examination involve?

_____

_____

_____

_____

(583)   **33.** A child with scoliosis who needs a spinal fusion has special needs related to immobilization. What is the appropriate nursing diagnosis?

_____

_____

(576-577) **34.** List the nursing care associated with immobility.

a. _____

b. _____

c. _____

d. _____

(583-584) **35.** A parent asks you for guidelines to help prevent sports injuries in a child who is in competitive sports. List four guidelines.

a. _____

b. _____

c. _____

d. _____

(584)   **36.** What is the treatment for shin splints?

_____

_____

(586)   **37.** When a nurse suspects child abuse he or she must _____

_____.

Student Name _____

THINKING CRITICALLY

1. Consider how a family is affected when a child is discharged from the hospital with a leg cast. Make a list of adaptations that may need to be made with regard to activities of daily living and family activities.

2. Nurses who care for abused children may have negative feelings toward the adult who abused the child. Examine your thoughts on this issue. Consider how supporting the adult will ultimately help the child.

CASE STUDY

1. Two-year-old Kimberly is admitted to the hospital with a fractured femur. She is placed in Bryant's traction.
   a. Kimberly's mother asks why this particular type of traction is used. How should the nurse reply?
   b. What particular areas of Kimberly's body would be assessed? Provide rationales.
   c. What are some diversional activities the nurse could plan for the child? Base the plan on knowledge of growth and development.

APPLYING KNOWLEDGE

1. While in the clinical area, care for a child in traction or in a body cast. Check your answers with an anatomy textbook.

2. Screen a 10-year-old girl for scoliosis.

3. Label the following bones on Figure 24-1 of the textbook.
   a. femur
   b. tibia
   c. fibula
   d. ulna
   e. radius
   f. coccyx
   g. clavicle
   h. humerus

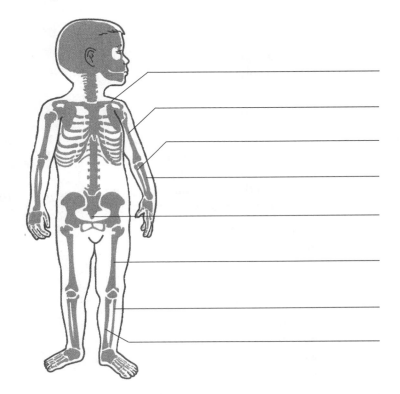

4. Help a child who is immobilized by a musculoskeletal condition plan his diet.

5. Give skin care to a child with skeletal traction.

6. Review teaching materials on cast care in your clinical facility.

REVIEW QUESTIONS

(579) **1.** One of the most common causes of death in a child with muscular dystrophy is

1. renal failure.
2. osteomyelitis.
3. cardiac failure.
4. liver disease.

(570) **2.** Which type of traction would the nurse expect to be used for a 20-month-old child who has a fractured femur?

1. Buck extension
2. Bryant's
3. Russell
4. ninety-ninety

(570) **3.** Damage to the epiphyseal plate in fractures involving a child can be serious because of

1. red blood cell production.
2. calcium storage.
3. bone growth.
4. bone healing.

(582) **4.** A child is referred to a physician after scoliosis screening. The physician plans to defer treatment and watch the child. You know that his curvature must be less than

1. 10 degrees.   2.   20 degrees.
3. 30 degrees.   4.   40 degrees.

(582) **5.** A child with suspected scoliosis might have

1. a prominent clavicle.
2. an expiratory wheeze.
3. asymmetry of the shoulders.
4. delayed breast development.

(579) **6.** Which of the following diseases is usually inherited as an X-linked disorder?

1. Legg-Calvé-Perthes disease
2. scoliosis
3. juvenile rheumatoid arthritis
4. Duchenne's muscular dystrophy

(579) **7.** Treatment of Legg-Calvé-Perthes disease consists of

1. complete bed rest.
2. no weight-bearing activity.
3. surgery.
4. ambulation-abduction casts or braces.

(570) **8.** Healing of a fracture in a child is

1. about the same as in an adult.
2. slower than in an adult.
3. faster than in an adult.

(578) **9.** Treatment of osteomyelitis includes the use of

1. steroids.
2. antibiotics.
3. traction.
4. hydrotherapy.

(580) **10.** The development of iridocyclitis is a complication of

1. Legg-Calvé-Perthes disease.
2. osteomyelitis.
3. juvenile rheumatoid arthritis.
4. scoliosis.

Student Name _____

(572) **11.** When caring for a child in Bryant's traction, the nurse should

1. remove the weights when bathing.
2. support the weights when the bed is moved.
3. position the child so the buttocks touch the bed.
4. position the child's legs at right angles to the body.

(580) **12.** A priority nursing diagnosis for an adolescent treated for osteosarcoma is

1. Risk for infection.
2. Post-trauma syndrome.
3. Disturbed body image.
4. Risk for trauma.

(579) **13.** Legg-Calvé-Perthes disease affects the

1. tip of the tibia.
2. shaft of the fibula.
3. head of the femur.
4. patella.

(581) **14.** The mother of an infant born with congenital torticollis is concerned that her child will always have limited neck motion. You know that

1. the child will always need to wear a neck brace.
2. surgery is the treatment of choice.
3. the condition will most likely resolve by 2–6 months.
4. there is nothing the mother can do to assist in the resolution of the condition.

(586) **15.** A child is being removed from the home of an abusive parent. The child is crying and a co-worker wonders if this could be a sign that the child was not abused. You know that the child

1. would not be crying if they had been abused in the home.
2. will mourn the loss of the family, even if there was abuse.
3. is seeking attention.
4. doesn't really understand what is happening.

(586) **16.** Which of the following statements by a mother might indicate future problems related to the care of a newborn infant?

1. "I am happy that my mother will be here for a few weeks. I feel overwhelmed caring for the baby and my other children."
2. "May I call you with questions? This is my first child and although I feel prepared, I am feeling frightened by the responsibility."
3. "The baby cries all the time. She doesn't seem to like me. I didn't think it would be like this. Sometimes I think she is just trying to irritate me."
4. "Our baby has colic. We are taking turns rocking her and getting up with her at night. When will we get a full night of sleep?"

CHAPTER 25

Student Name _____

The Child with a Respiratory or Cardiovascular Disorder

Answer Key: Textbook page references are provided as a guide for answering these questions. A complete answer key was provided for your instructor.

LEARNING ACTIVITIES

1. Match the terms in the left column with their definitions on the right (a–e).

(609) _____ clubbing   a. difficult swallowing
                       b. harsh, high-pitched sound on inspiration

(594) _____ stridor   c. asthma attack that is not responsive to drugs
                       d. increased red blood cells

(621) _____ polycythemia   e. compensatory response indicating a chronic lack of oxygen

(607) _____ status asthmaticus

(594) _____ dysphagia

(591) **2.** List six of the more common procedures used to diagnose respiratory conditions.

     a. _____

     b. _____

     c. _____

     d. _____

     e. _____

     f. _____

(591) **3.** The common cold is also known as _____.

(592-594) **4.** List five measures that can relieve the symptoms of the common cold.

    a. _____

    b. _____

    c. _____

    d. _____

    e. _____

(594) **5.** Define the term *croup*.

_____

_____

_____

(595) **6.** Describe the clinical course of laryngotracheobronchitis.

_____

_____

_____

_____

_____

(595) **7.** What advice would you give a parent about home care of a child with croup?

_____

_____

_____

_____

_____

(596) **8.** If epiglottitis is suspected, what nursing responsibility must be instituted?

_____

(596) **9.** The treatment of choice for a child with epiglottitis is a _____

or _____.

Student Name _____

(597) **10.** List the common signs and symptoms of bronchiolitis.

a. _____

b. _____

c. _____

d. _____

(597) **11.** What position facilitates breathing for the infant with bronchiolitis?

_____

(597) **12.** Respiratory syncytial virus (RSV) is spread by _____.

(597) **13.** RSV can survive for more than _____ hours on countertops, tissues, and soap.

(597) **14.** The priority nursing diagnosis for an infant hospitalized with RSV infection is

_____.

(598) **15.** List four of the possible signs of respiratory distress.

a. _____

b. _____

c. _____

d. _____

(599) **16.** What are some of the common signs and symptoms of pneumonia?

a. _____

b. _____

c. _____

d. _____

(599) **17.** The removal of the tonsils and adenoids should wait until the child is at least

_____ years of age.

(599-600) **18.** What signs and symptoms are indicative of bleeding in the postoperative tonsillectomy patient?

a. _____

b. _____

c. _____

d. _____

(602) **19.** Describe the pathologic changes that take place in asthma.

_____

_____

_____

_____

_____

(603) **20.** List five signs and symptoms of asthma.

a. _____

b. _____

c. _____

d. _____

e. _____

(603-304) **21.** Name three bronchodilators used in the management of asthma.

a. _____

b. _____

c. _____

(604-605) **22.** Name three antiinflammatory medications used in the management of asthma.

a. _____

b. _____

c. _____

Student Name_____

(605)   **23.**   What would the nurse teach the family of a child with asthma about controlling allergens in the child's bedroom?

_____

_____

_____

_____

(606)   **24.**   Why should a child with asthma use a spacer with a metered dose inhaler?

_____

(608)   **25.**   Cystic fibrosis is an _____ _____ disease. That means

_____ parent(s) carry the gene for the disease.

(608)   **26.**   Describe how cystic fibrosis affects the child's respiratory system.

_____

_____

_____

_____

(608)   **27.**   Describe the stools of a child with cystic fibrosis.

_____

(609)   **28.**   What physiologic changes take place in the pancreas of a child with cystic fibrosis?

_____

_____

_____

(609)   **29.**   A _____ is the test of choice for

diagnosing cystic fibrosis.

(609-614) **30.** List three ways respiratory complications can be decreased in patients with cystic fibrosis.

a. _____

_____

b. _____

_____

c. _____

_____

(609-614) **31.** Discharge teaching of a child with cystic fibrosis should include instructions about:

a. _____

b. _____

c. _____

d. _____

e. _____

f. _____

(614) **32.** Children with cystic fibrosis should receive which vitamin supplements?

_____

(615) **33.** One of the greatest challenges for the family and the child who is technology-dependent is to

maintain optimum _____ and _____.

(616) **34.** The nurse teaches parents to place infants in the _____ position for sleep.

This measure reduces the risk of _____.

(616) **35.** List five signs that indicate an infant may have a congenital heart defect.

a. _____

b. _____

c. _____

d. _____

e. _____

*① List 5 signs that indicate an infant may have a congenital heart defect?   pg 597 text

239

Student Name _____

● (616) 36. _____ are the leading cause of death
among the congenital anomalies during the first year of life.

(617) 37. Heart defects can be classified as lesions that:

    a. _____

    b. _____

    c. _____

38. Match the types of heart defects on the left with their definitions on the right (a–d).

(619)   _____ ventricular septal defect   a. narrowing of the aortic arch or the descend-
ing aorta

(620)   _____ coarctation of the aorta   b. opening between the right and left ventricles

                                                    c. failure of the ductus arteriosus to close

(618)   _____ atrial septal defect   d. opening between left and right atria

(620)   _____ patent ductus arteriosus

● (618) 39. In a child with an atrial septal defect, you would expect _____

_____ blood to move from the

_____ atrium to the _____ atrium. The

defect causes a _____ to _____ shunting of blood.

(620) 40. What is the classic sign of coarctation of the aorta?

_____

_____

(618) 41. Why are prophylactic antibiotics given to children with ventricular septal defects?

✳ _____

_____

(620) 42. List the signs and symptoms of patent ductus arteriosus.

    a. _____

✳   b. _____

●   c. _____

    d. _____

(620-621) **43.** Describe the four defects that make up tetralogy of Fallot.

a. _____

b. _____

c. _____

d. _____

(621) **44.** List the signs and symptoms of tetralogy of Fallot.

a. _____

b. _____

c. _____

d. _____

e. _____

f. _____

g. _____

(621) **45.** Explain why polycythemia develops in children with heart defects.

_____

_____

(623) **46.** List four signs and symptoms of congestive heart failure. PG 602

a. _____

b. _____

c. _____

d. _____

(623) **47.** Respirations over _____ breaths/minute in a newborn at rest indicate distress.

(623-624) **48.** Nursing goals when caring for a child with a heart defect include: PG 602

a. _____

b. _____

c. _____

Student Name _____

d. _____

e. _____

f. _____

(624) **49.** List three nursing actions you could take to conserve the energy of a child with a heart defect.

a. _____

_____

b. _____

_____

c. _____

_____

(624) **50.** Children receiving diuretics must have their serum _____ monitored closely.

(624) **51.** List four foods high in potassium.

a. _____

b. _____

c. _____

d. _____

_____

(624) **52.** List the signs and symptoms of digitalis toxicity.

a. _____

b. _____

c. _____

d. _____

e. _____

(625)   **53.**   What are the classic symptoms of rheumatic fever?

    a.   _____

    b.   _____

    c.   _____

    d.   _____

(627)   **54.**   Rheumatic fever can be avoided by identification of _____

    infections and treatment with _____.

(627)   **55.**   What advice would you give an adolescent who shows a consistently high blood pressure reading?

    _____

(628)   **56.**   Kawasaki's disease causes _____ of the vessels in the

    cardiovascular system, which can result in _____.

(628)   **57.**   Name three medications that may be used in the treatment of Kawasaki's disease.

    a.   _____

    b.   _____

    c.   _____

THINKING CRITICALLY

    1.   You are caring for a 1-month-old infant with a ventricular septal defect who is in congestive heart failure. When you measured the infant's apical heart rate, before his 8:00 AM dose of Lanoxin, it was 112 bpm. Should you administer the Lanoxin?

    2.   Plan for the discharge of a child newly diagnosed with cystic fibrosis. Include diet, medication, respiratory care, and psychologic care of the child and the parents.

    3.   Develop a plan of care for a child with a congenital heart defect. Incorporate into the plan the child's physiologic and psychologic needs.

Student Name _____

CASE STUDIES

1. Six-year-old Jasmine is admitted to the hospital with a diagnosis of asthma. She is restless, has difficulty breathing, and is wheezing. She has numerous allergies.
   a. Jasmine relates that she has been taking allergy shots and they have removed many of the objects she is allergic to from their home. Explain each of these methods of allergy treatment.
   b. What position should Jasmine assume to decrease respiratory distress?
   c. The physician wants Jasmine to have increased fluid intake. What liquids should be encouraged and which should be avoided?
   d. Jasmine wants to participate in the swim team at school. What should the nurse tell her about asthma and exercise?

2. Alicia, an 8-year-old child, is admitted to the hospital with cystic fibrosis. She has a history of chronic pulmonary and sinus problems.
   a. Alicia takes an oral pancreatic enzyme. When should she take this medication?
   b. Alicia has extensive lung disease. What measures would improve respiration?
   c. What type of diet would be ordered for Alicia?
   d. Alicia's appetite has markedly decreased. What can be done to increase her intake?

APPLYING KNOWLEDGE

1. Observe a cardiac catheterization in the clinical area.

2. Care for a child with cardiac disease.

3. Care for a child who has had cardiac surgery.

4. Care for a child in an oxygen tent who has a respiratory disease.

5. Care for a child who has had a tonsillectomy.

6. Admit a child to the unit who has asthma.

7. Teach a child with cystic fibrosis about respiratory care and diet.

8. Become certified in pediatric CPR.

9. While in the clinical area, locate the unit's emergency cart and review the contents.

REVIEW QUESTIONS

(619) **1.** The most common heart defect in children is

1. ventricular septal defect.
2. coarctation of the aorta.
3. atrial septal defect.
4. patent ductus arteriosus.

(624) **2.** The best method of feeding infants with heart defects is to

1. space feedings at least every 3–4 hours.
2. give frequent, large feedings.
3. feed intravenously.
4. feed smaller amounts more frequently.

(624) **3.** If the pulse of a newborn is below _____ bpm, digitalis is withheld.

1. 120   2. 110
3. 100   4. 90

(624) **4.** Signs and symptoms of digitoxin toxicity include

1. retention of water.
2. diarrhea.
3. nausea and vomiting.
4. headaches.

(624) **5.** When a child is on diuretics, it is the nurse's responsibility to

1. withhold fluids.
2. monitor serum electrolyte levels.
3. place on seizure precautions.
4. check the dosage with another nurse before giving.

(627) **6.** A child who is hypertensive is identified during routine screening. The child should be

1. placed on diuretics.
2. placed on beta-adrenergic blockers.
3. put on an exercise and diet program.
4. scheduled for two more blood pressure readings.

(621) **7.** An infant with tetralogy of Fallot becomes hypercyanotic. The nurse would place the infant in the _____ position.

1. high Fowler's
2. Trendelenburg
3. side-lying
4. knee-chest

(597) **8.** An appropriate treatment for a child with bronchiolitis is

1. isolation.
2. increased fluids.
3. antihistamines.
4. increased solids.

(599) **9.** The best liquid to give to a child who has had a tonsillectomy is

1. orange juice.
2. milk.
3. hot chocolate.
4. a popsicle.

(614) **10.** A child with cystic fibrosis should be placed on a diet that is

1. high calorie, high protein, moderate fat.
2. high calorie, low protein, low fat.
3. low calorie, high protein, low fat.
4. high calorie, low protein, moderate fat.

(595) **11.** Children with croup are placed in an environment of high humidity in order to

1. decrease the possibility of a bacterial infection.
2. increase the child's appetite.
3. liquefy secretions.
4. decrease body temperature.

Student Name _____

(596) **12.** If a child is suspected of having epiglottitis, the nurse should

1. avoid examination of the pharynx.
2. force fluids.
3. place the child on the right side.
4. place the child in isolation.

(599) **13.** Which of the following could indicate a postoperative emergency in a tonsillectomy patient?

1. sore throat
2. vomiting pink-tinged blood
3. low-grade fever
4. frequent swallowing

(606) **14.** The child with asthma should be instructed to

1. avoid exercise.
2. avoid hot liquids.
3. identify early signs of an asthma attack.
4. decrease the amount of liquids taken after 6:00 PM.

(616) **15.** A child with a congenital heart abnormality would most likely experience

1. difficulty feeding.
2. difficulty sleeping.
3. normal weight gain.
4. decreased blood pressure.

(605) **16.** Fluids offered to the child with asthma should not be too cold because cold fluids may

1. increase the chance of dehydration.
2. trigger reflex bronchospasm.
3. cause nausea and vomiting.
4. increase mucus.

(614) **17.** Which medication is not useful when a child is experiencing an asthma attack?

1. albuterol
2. cromolyn sodium
3. corticosteroids
4. theophylline

(620) **18.** A congenital heart defect that results in decreased pulmonary blood flow is

1. atrial septal defect.
2. aortic stenosis.
3. tetralogy of Fallot.
4. patent ductus arteriosus.

CROSSWORD PUZZLE

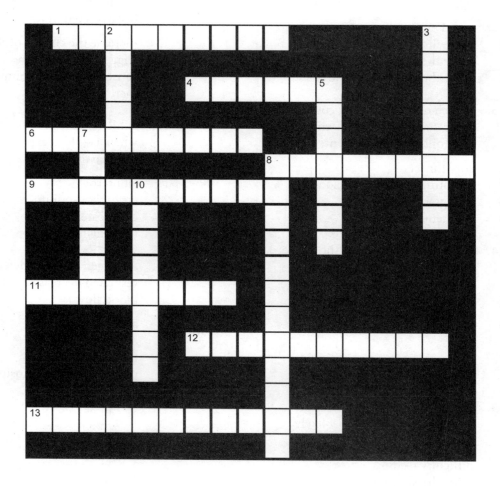

Across

(597)	1.	Increased respiratory rate
(591)	4.	A cold
(594)	6.	Painful swallowing
(620)	8.	Obstruction to blood flow caused by narrowing of a vessel
(591)	9.	Prevents the alveoli from collapsing during respiration after birth
(625)	11.	Inflammation of the heart
(602)	12.	Increased airway responsiveness in asthma is intermittent or _____
(621)	13.	Increased number of red blood cells

Down

(594)	2.	General term applied to a number of conditions with symptoms of a brassy cough and varying degrees of stridor
(609)	3.	Compensatory response to chronic lack of oxygen
(598)	5.	Air sacs in the lungs
(594)	7.	Harsh, high-pitched sound heard on inspiration
(623)	8.	Amount of blood ejected during one heart contraction
(622)	10.	Heart disease occurring after birth

CHAPTER 26

The Child with a Condition of the Blood, Blood-Forming Organs, or Lymphatic System

Answer Key: Textbook page references are provided as a guide for answering these questions. A complete answer key was provided for your instructor.

LEARNING ACTIVITIES

1. Match the terms in the left column with their definitions on the right (a–g).

(643)	_____ alopecia	a. red blood cells (RBCs)
		b. pinpoint hemorrhagic spots beneath the skin
(631)	_____ erythrocytes	c. white blood cells (WBCs)
		d. platelets
(637)	_____ hemarthrosis	e. hemorrhage into a joint cavity
		f. loss of hair
(630)	_____ leukocytes	g. larger hemorrhagic spots in the skin
(632)	_____ petechiae	
(632)	_____ purpura	
(632)	_____ thrombocytes	

(632) **2.** State the functions of the following blood components.

a. leukocytes _____

b. erythrocytes _____

c. thrombocytes _____

(633) **3.** List the causes of iron deficiency anemia.

a. _____

b. _____

c. _____

d. _____

(635)   **4.**   List four food sources with high iron content.

        a. _____

        b. _____

        c. _____

        d. _____

(634)   **5.**   List the major signs and symptoms of iron-deficiency anemia.

        a. _____

        b. _____

        c. _____

        d. _____

(634)   **6.**   Infants should be screened for iron-deficiency anemia at _____ and _____ months of age.

(634)   **7.**   What instructions would you give to a parent about administering an iron supplement to a toddler?

        _____

        _____

        _____

(634)   **8.**   Describe the stools of a young child receiving an iron supplement.

        _____

(634)   **9.**   What should the nurse tell a parent about formula and milk intake during the first year of life?

        _____

        _____

        _____

(634)   **10.**   Sickle cell disease is most prevalent in the _____

        _____ population.

Student Name_____

● *(634)* **11.** List four factors that might trigger a sickle cell crisis.

   a. _____

   b. _____

   c. _____

   d. _____

(636) **12.** Explain the difference between sickle cell trait and sickle cell disease.

_____

_____

_____

_____

(636) **13.** The child with sickle cell disease inherits the abnormality from _____

_____.

● *(638)* **14.** List the types of sickle cell crises.

   a. _____

   b. _____

   c. _____

   d. _____

(636) **15.** List three of the possible signs and symptoms of a sickle cell crisis.

   a. _____

   b. _____

   c. _____

(636) **16.** What is the most common test used to screen for sickle cell disease?

_____

●

(637) **17.** Patient-controlled analgesia can be used for the child over _____ years of age to manage pain caused by sickle cell crisis.

(637) **18.** List two priority goals when caring for a child with sickle cell disease.

a. _____

b. _____

(639) **19.** The mainstay of treatment for thalassemia major is _____

_____.

(639) **20.** Children with thalassemia major develop _____ as a result of treatment.

(640) **21.** Hemophilia is inherited as a _____trait.

(640) **22.** Hemophilia A is caused by a deficiency of _____.

(640) **23.** A classic symptom of hemophilia is _____,

which is a hemorrhage into a _____.

(640) **24.** The principal therapy for hemophilia is to prevent _____ by replacing the missing factor.

(640) **25.** _____ is a nasal spray that can stop bleeding and may be the treatment of choice for mild cases of hemophilia.

(641) **26.** When bleeding occurs in a child with hemophilia, the traditional approach is to include

_____, _____, _____

and _____.

(641) **27.** Describe the clinical manifestations of idiopathic thrombocytopenic purpura (ITP).

_____

_____

_____

_____

(642) **28.** The most common form of childhood cancer is _____.

Student Name_____

(642)   **29.**   Leukemia results in the uncontrolled growth of _____

_____.

(642)   **30.**   Explain the pathologic changes that take place when a child has leukemia.

_____

_____

_____

(642)   **31.**   List seven of the possible presenting signs and symptoms of leukemia.

a.   _____

b.   _____

c.   _____

d.   _____

e.   _____

f.   _____

g.   _____

(643)   **32.**   List the five phases of treatment of leukemia.

a.   _____

b.   _____

c.   _____

d.   _____

e.   _____

(643)   **33.**   List some of the common side effects of chemotherapy.

a.   _____

b.   _____

c.   _____

d.   _____

e.   _____

(644) **34.** Identify three nursing interventions appropriate for a 10-year-old girl who is worried about alopecia associated with chemotherapy.

a. _____

b. _____

c. _____

(644) **35.** List five signs of a transfusion reaction.

a. _____

b. _____

c. _____

d. _____

e. _____

(644) **36.** If a child showed signs of a transfusion reaction, the nurse's initial action would be to

_____.

Answer as either true (T) or false (F).

(645) **37.** Hodgkin's disease is a malignancy of the lymph system. _____

(645) **38.** The presenting sign of Hodgkin's disease is usually pain in the neck and shoulders. _____

(645) **39.** The treatment of Hodgkin's disease involves chemotherapy and radiation therapy. _____

(645) **40.** Following a splenectomy, the child faces the long-term risk of serious _____.

(651) **41.** Describe the preschooler's response to the death of a sibling.

_____

(651) **42.** The primary fear of dying children younger than 5 years of age is

_____.

(651) **43.** Children develop an understanding of death as permanent around age

_____ years.

Student Name_____

THINKING CRITICALLY

1. Develop a nursing care plan for a child with sickle cell disease experiencing a vaso-occlusive crisis.

2. Review the genetic implications of sickle cell disease by answering the following questions:

   Results of hemoglobin electrophoresis show that an infant has sickle cell anemia. The infant's parents desire to have several more children. When both parents have the sickle cell trait, what are the chances that:
   a. a child will have sickle cell anemia?
   b. a child will carry the sickle cell trait?
   c. a child will have neither the disease nor the trait?
   d. Will the child's gender affect whether the child has the disease? Why or why not?

3. Review the genetic implications of hemophilia when a mother is a carrier of the hemophilia gene and the father does not have the disease.
   a. What are the chances that a son will have the disease?
   b. What are the chances that a daughter will be a carrier?
   c. Why does the child's gender affect whether he or she can manifest this disease?

CASE STUDY

1. Lauren, a 5-year-old girl, is hospitalized with acute lymphocytic leukemia (ALL). She is receiving chemotherapy and has been placed in a private room.
   a. What special precautions should be taken with a child who is immune-suppressed?
   b. Lauren develops ulcerations in her mouth. What can the nurse do to relieve discomfort and promote healing of the oral mucosa?
   c. Lauren is to receive a unit of packed red blood cells. For what signs and symptoms of a reaction should the nurse observe and what action would be taken if a reaction occurred?

APPLYING KNOWLEDGE

1. While in the clinical area, care for a child who has cancer and is receiving chemotherapy.

2. While in the clinical area, care for a child who is in sickle cell crisis.

3. Observe a bone marrow aspiration being performed.

4. Speak with a pediatric nurse who works with children who have cancer about her feelings when a child dies.

5. Visit the Ronald McDonald House in your city. Discuss with your classmates the setting and the services.

6. Discuss with your classmates your feelings when you must cause discomfort to a child in order to help him or her.

7. Develop a family education sheet on preventing iron deficiency anemia.

REVIEW QUESTIONS

(651)   **1.**   By what age do children realize that death is final and permanent?

1.   3 years   2.   5 years
3.   7 years   4.   10 years

(634)   **2.**   Iron absorption is increased by taking it with

1.   orange juice.
2.   cereal.
3.   milk.
4.   eggs.

(634)   **3.**   It is recommended that iron-fortified formula be given to infants through age

1.   3 months.   2.   6 months.
3.   9 months.   4.   12 months.

(640)   **4.**   Which of the following presents the greatest risk to the child with hemophilia?

1.   hematuria
2.   hemarthrosis
3.   intracranial bleeding
4.   anemia

(641)   **5.**   Signs and symptoms that might indicate that a child has idiopathic thrombocytopenic purpura include

1.   headaches and hematuria.
2.   anemia and purpura.
3.   petechiae and purpura.
4.   hematuria and petechiae.

(642)   **6.**   The diagnostic test that confirms a diagnosis of leukemia is a(n)

1.   spinal tap.
2.   bone marrow aspiration.
3.   complete blood count.
4.   x-ray of the bones.

(643)   **7.**   When caring for a child on steroid therapy, it is important to seek immediate medical attention if the child

1.   vomits.
2.   develops a fever.
3.   skips a meal.
4.   gains weight.

(645)   **8.**   Children with Hodgkin's disease usually present with a(n)

1.   rapid weight loss.
2.   painless cervical neck lump.
3.   enlarged abdomen.
4.   high fever.

(641)   **9.**   Children with hemophilia should avoid

1.   swimming.
2.   salicylates.
3.   citrus fruits.
4.   analgesics.

(636)   **10.** Children with sickle cell trait

1.   have a 10% chance of developing the disease.
2.   have a 25% chance of developing the disease.
3.   have a 50% chance of developing the disease.
4.   will not develop the disease.

(636-637) **11.** An appropriate nursing intervention for the child admitted to the hospital in sickle cell crisis would be to

1.   apply ice to painful areas.
2.   encourage the child to ambulate.
3.   provide foods high in iron at meals.
4.   monitor the child's response to analgesics.

Student Name _____

(641) **12.** Immediate nursing care of a child with hemophilia who has hemarthrosis includes

1. application of heat.
2. active and passive range-of-motion exercises.
3. immobilization of the area.
4. withholding factor VIII.

(641) **13.** The greatest concern of a nurse caring for a child with ITP is

1. noncompliance with aspirin therapy.
2. a reaction to platelets.
3. injuries that might initiate bleeding.
4. development of a secondary bacterial infection.

(644) **14.** Anxiety can be decreased in both the family and the child who has cancer by

1. not telling the child that he or she has cancer.
2. explaining all procedures before they are done.
3. placing the child with an older child who has the same diagnosis.
4. discouraging the child and parents from discussing the issue of death.

(643) **15.** A common childhood disease that can have devastating effects on an immune-suppressed child is

1. measles.
2. chickenpox.
3. rubella.
4. nasopharyngitis.

(647-648) **16.** Nursing care of an adolescent with cancer who is refusing to cooperate with treatment should include

1. asking the parents to make the adolescent cooperate.
2. allowing the adolescent to make some choices.
3. withholding favorite foods until the behavior changes.
4. restricting visitors until the behavior is modified.

(644) **17.** A child with cancer refuses mouth care. The best response is

1. "We can wait until the next time when you are not so uncomfortable."
2. "I will see if the doctor will let us stop doing mouth care."
3. "If you will cooperate this time, we can skip mouth care later today."
4. "Although I know it is uncomfortable, we must do this to prevent even more problems in your mouth."

CROSSWORD PUZZLE

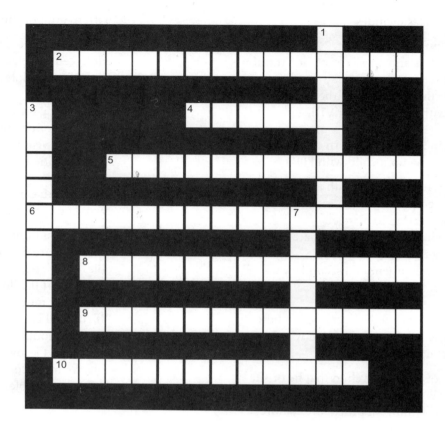

Across

(631)   2.   Regulates the rate of RBC production

(633)   4.   A reduction in the size of RBCs or in amount of circulating hemoglobin

(640)   5.   Bleeding into a joint cavity

(632)   6.   Enlargement of lymph nodes

(637)   8.   Deposit of iron into organs and tissues of the body

(638)   9.   Type of sickle cell crisis caused by obstruction to blood flow by abnormally shaped cells

(632)   10.   Enlargement of the spleen

Down

(641)   1.   Raised ecchymosis

(641)   3.   A physician who specializes in treating cancer

(632)   7.   Groups of adjoining petechiae

CHAPTER

27 The Child with a Gastrointestinal Condition

Answer Key: Textbook page references are provided as a guide for answering these questions. A complete answer key was provided for your instructor.

LEARNING ACTIVITIES

1. Match the terms in the left column with their definitions on the right (a–g).

(670) _____ homeostasis

(663) _____ incarcerated

(663) _____ inguinal hernia

(680) _____ pica

(658) _____ projectile vomiting

(659) _____ pyloromyotomy

(680) _____ plumbism

a. protrusion of part of the intestine through the umbilical ring
b. constricted hernia
c. eating nonfood items
d. operation to correct pyloric stenosis
e. state of equilibrium of the body
f. vomiting in which the stomach contents are forcibly ejected
g. lead poisoning

(656) **2.** List four of the possible common tests used to diagnose gastrointestinal disorders.

a. _____

b. _____

c. _____

d. _____

(658) **3.** The infant with tracheoesophageal fistula will _____ and

_____ when the first feeding is given.

(658) **4.** Describe the usual progression of signs and symptoms in a child with pyloric stenosis.

_____

_____

_____

_____

(658) **5.** A complication of the vomiting associated with pyloric stenosis is

_____.

(659) **6.** Describe the progression of feeding after postoperative correction of pyloric stenosis.

_____

_____

_____

_____

_____

(659) **7.** Celiac disease is the leading _____ problem in children.

(660) **8.** Gluten is found in _____, _____, _____, and

_____.

(660) **9.** Stools in the child with celiac disease are _____, _____,

and _____.

(661) **10.** The earliest sign of Hirschsprung's disease is failure to pass meconium stools within

_____ to _____ hours after birth.

(662) **11.** Hirschsprung's disease is treated _____. It may be necessary for

the infant to have a _____ temporarily.

Student Name_____

(662) **12.** Tap water enemas are never given to children because they can lead to

_____ and _____

(662) **13.** Describe the initial onset of intussusception.

_____

_____

_____

(662) **14.** Treatment of choice for intussusception is reduction through the use of a

_____.

(663) **15.** The most common congenital malformation of the gastrointestinal tract is

_____.

(663) **16.** Surgical repair of a hernia is called a _____

_____.

(663) **17.** Name the priority concerns when an infant has diarrhea.

a. _____

b. _____

(663) **18.** Nursing interventions related to gastroenteritis focus on:

a. _____

b. _____

c. _____

(664) **19.** Persistent vomiting can result in _____

and _____.

(664) **20.** To prevent aspiration of vomitus after feeding, a child should be placed in what position?

_____

(664) **21.** What would be included in the nurse's documentation for a child who is vomiting?

a. _____

b. _____

c. _____

d. _____

e. _____

f. _____

g. _____

(665) **22.** After a feeding, an infant with gastroesophageal reflux disease should be placed in which position?

_____

(666) **23.** Signs and symptoms of dehydration in the infant include:

a. _____

b. _____

c. _____

d. _____

(666) **24.** A 6-year-old child has mild diarrhea. How would the nurse advise the child's parents about fluid and food intake?

_____

(666) **25.** Name three high-fiber foods to recommend to an older child who is experiencing constipation.

a. _____

b. _____

c. _____

(666) **26.** In children under age 2, a greater percentage of body water is contained in the

_____ compartment.

Student Name _____

(671) **27.** _____ is the greatest
threat to life in isotonic dehydration.

(637) **28.** Failure to thrive (FTT) describes infants and children who _____

_____.

(674) **29.** Kwashiorkor results from a severe deficiency of _____ in the
child's diet.

(675) **30.** List three signs and symptoms of rickets.

  a. _____

  b. _____

  c. _____

(675) **31.** The decrease of incidence of rickets in the world is attributed to

_____.

(675) **32.** Scurvy results from a deficiency of foods containing _____ in

the diet. To prevent scurvy, the nurse would encourage parents to include

_____ and

_____ in the child's diet.

Answer as either true (T) or false (F).

(675) **33.** Vomiting begins before abdominal pain with appendicitis. _____

(675) **34.** Fever is a reliable sign of appendicitis in children. _____

(675) **35.** Abdominal pain associated with appendicitis is localized in the right lower quadrant. _____

(675) **36.** The child with appendicitis may exhibit guarding and rebound tenderness when the nurse
performs an abdominal assessment. _____

(676) **37.** How is Nystatin applied to the mouth of a child with thrush?

_____

(676) **38.** Explain how pinworm infestation is spread.

_____

_____

_____

_____

(676) **39.** What is the most common sign of pinworms?

_____

(676) **40.** Describe the treatment of pinworms.

_____

_____

_____

_____

_____

(677) **41.** The goals in the treatment of poisoning are:

a. _____

b. _____

c. _____

d. _____

(677) **42.** Ipecac should not be used if the child ingested _____,

_____, _____, and

_____, or if the child is not

_____.

(677) **43.** Activated charcoal should not be given with _____ because it will neutralize both, rendering both ineffective in the treatment of poisoning.

(678) **44.** An overdose of acetaminophen can result in _____ damage.

Student Name _____

(680)   **45.**   The primary source of lead poisoning is _____.

(681)   **46.**   Lead poisoning can have a lasting effect on the _____ system.

           47.   Match each type of dehydration with its definition (a–c).

(671)   _____ hypotonic   a.   loss of more electrolytes than water

                                                    b.   loss of equal amounts of water and electro-

(671)   _____ hypertonic   lytes

                                                    c.   loss of more water than electrolytes

(671)   _____ isotonic

THINKING CRITICALLY

    1.   You are speaking to a parent whose child has mild diarrhea. The parent explains that she has been giving the child a BRAT diet. Is this an appropriate intervention? If not, what will you recommend for this child?

    2.   You are caring for a child who drank a poisonous substance. What feelings might the child's parents be having? How can you assist the parents?

CASE STUDY

    1.   Six-month-old Amber is diagnosed as failing to thrive. Amber's mother is a single parent who does not work outside the home. Neighbors report that they often hear Amber crying and that her mother seldom holds her. They also report that Amber's mother has related to them that being a mother is not what she thought it would be.
       a.   List some of the signs of failure to thrive.
       b.   What treatment might be implemented?
       c.   How would you involve Amber's mother in her care?
       d.   Discuss your feelings toward parents who neglect their children.

APPLYING KNOWLEDGE

    1.   Observe an endoscopy.

2.   Use Figure 27-1 in the textbook to label the following.

    a.   esophagus
    b.   stomach
    c.   pancreas
    d.   liver
    e.   gallbladder
    f.   small intestine
    g.   large intestine
    h.   rectum

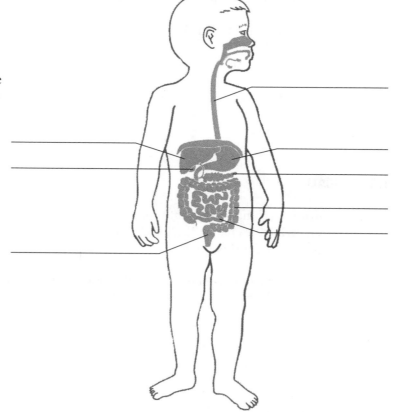

3.   Develop a teaching plan related to poison prevention.

4.   Develop a teaching plan related to caring for a child with diarrhea.

REVIEW QUESTIONS

(656)   **1.**   The upper GI tract can be visualized through

    1.   colonoscopy.
    2.   sigmoidoscopy.
    3.   endoscopy.
    4.   proctoscopy.

(673)   **2.**   Children with failure to thrive fall below the _____ percentile on growth charts.

    1.   3rd
    2.   6th
    3.   10th
    4.   15th

(674)   **3.**   Which approach might best support maternal attachment when caring for a child with failure to thrive?

    1.   Point out areas where the mother needs improvement.
    2.   Send the mother to a parenting class.
    3.   Role-model appropriate care of the child.
    4.   Leave the room when the mother visits.

Student Name _____

(676) **4.** Signs and symptoms of pinworms are

1. diarrhea, itching, and fever.
2. nausea, vomiting, and itching.
3. nausea, vomiting, and weight loss.
4. itching, irritability, and restlessness.

(662) **5.** Children with intussusception may have bowel movements containing blood and mucus and no feces. These are called

1. currant-jelly stools.
2. mucoid stools.
3. steatorrhea.
4. occult blood stools.

(669) **6.** A newborn's total body weight is about _____ water.

1. 77%   2. 65%
3. 55%   4. 45%

(672) **7.** Before potassium is added to an IV, the nurse should

1. take a baseline blood pressure.
2. darken the room.
3. establish that the child is voiding.
4. place the child on a cardiac monitor.

(671) **8.** The greatest threat to life in isotonic dehydration is

1. hypervolemic shock.
2. hypovolemic shock.
3. respiratory acidosis.
4. respiratory alkalosis.

(658) **9.** A classic sign of pyloric stenosis is

1. constipation.
2. projectile vomiting.
3. diarrhea.
4. anorexia.

(677) **10.** When a child has pinworms, the nurse knows that

1. it is a sign of poor hygiene.
2. the child will be hospitalized.
3. any family member with symptoms should be treated.
4. a warm stool specimen is sent to the lab.

(665) **11.** Treatment of gastroesophageal reflux disease includes

1. feeding half-strength formula.
2. positioning in an infant seat after feeding.
3. increasing the time between feedings.
4. placing the infant prone with the head elevated after feeding.

(661) **12.** The earliest sign of Hirschsprung's disease is

1. failure to pass meconium stools.
2. chronic constipation of the newborn.
3. chronic diarrhea of the newborn.
4. ribbon-like stools.

(679) **13.** The organ damaged by acetaminophen poisoning is the

1. gallbladder.
2. pancreas.
3. liver.
4. stomach.

(677) **14.** Infants are more susceptible to accidental ingestion of nonfood objects because they

1. are often left unattended.
2. are curious.
3. are constantly hungry.
4. want the attention.

(658) **15.** The nurse was giving a newborn her first feeding when the baby started coughing and choking. This is indicative of which condition?

1. celiac disease
2. enterocolitis
3. tracheoesophageal atresia
4. pyloric stenosis

(675) **16.** A child appears apathetic and weak. His growth is below normal for his age. There is a white streak in the child's hair. The nurse recognizes these signs as characteristic of

1. rickets
2. scurvy
3. gastroesophageal reflux
4. kwashiorkor

CHAPTER

28 The Child with a Genitourinary Condition

Answer Key: Textbook page references are provided as a guide for answering these questions. A complete answer key was provided for your instructor.

LEARNING ACTIVITIES

1.   Match the terms in the left column with their definitions on the right (a–j).

(688)   _____ cystitis

(684)   _____ encopresis

(686)   _____ enuresis

(690)   _____ glomeruli

(687)   _____ hypospadias

(686)   _____ phimosis

(688)   _____ pyelonephritis

(686)   _____ urgency

(688)   _____ urethritis

(689)   _____ vesicoureteral reflux

a.   backward flow of urine into the ureters
b.   abnormal number of voidings in a short period of time
c.   inflammation of the bladder
d.   infection of the kidney substance and pelvis
e.   infection of the ureters
f.   uncontrolled voiding after bladder control has been established
g.   narrowing of the preputial opening of the foreskin
h.   the working units of the kidney
i.   congenital defect in which the urinary meatus is not at the end of the penis but on the lower shaft
j.   fecal soiling beyond 4 years of age

(683)   **2.**   The functional unit of the kidney is the _____.

(686)   **3.**   List five tests used to determine the cause of urinary dysfunction.

         a.   _____

         b.   _____

         c.   _____

         d.   _____

         e.   _____

Answer as either true (T) or false (F).

(686)   **4.**   Phimosis is normal in newborn males and usually disappears by the time a boy is 3 years old. _____

(687)   **5.**   The optimal time for surgical repair of hypospadias and epispadias is in the late preschool period. _____

(688)   **6.**   Surgical repair of exstrophy of the bladder is done in the first 2 days of life. _____

(688)   **7.**   Distention of the renal pelvis due to an obstruction is referred to as

_____.

(688-689) **8.**   List four of the possible reasons why urinary tract infections are more common in girls than in boys.

   a.   _____

   b.   _____

   c.   _____

   d.   _____

(689)   **9.**   Compare the signs and symptoms of a urinary tract infection in infants with those in older children.

	Infant	*Older Child*
a.	_____	_____
b.	_____	_____
c.	_____	_____
d.	_____	_____

(689)   **10.**   What laboratory test is done to confirm a diagnosis of urinary tract infection?

_____

(689)   **11.**   What type of medication is used to treat a urinary tract infection in a 4-year-old child?

_____

(690)   **12.**   The characteristic sign of nephrotic syndrome is _____.

Student Name _____

(690) **13.** Edema associated with nephrotic syndrome usually occurs first around the

_____ and _____.

(690) **14.** The nurse would expect a urinalysis of a child with nephrotic syndrome to reveal massive

_____.

(690) **15.** What is the treatment of choice for nephrosis?

_____

(690) **16.** List three types of skin care that might be given to a child with nephrotic syndrome.

a. _____

b. _____

c. _____

(690, 692) **17.** List three nursing interventions used with a child who is anorexic secondary to nephrosis.

a. _____

b. _____

c. _____

(692) **18.** When observing the urine of a child with nephrosis, the nurse should note:

a. _____

b. _____

c. _____

d. _____

(693) **19.** Acute glomerulonephritis is thought to be a(n) _____

_____ reaction caused by _____

_____.

(693-694) **20.** List four nursing interventions that would be appropriate for the child who has acute glomerulonephritis.

    a. _____

    b. _____

    c. _____

    d. _____

(694) **21.** What organ is affected by Wilms' tumor? _____

(694) **22.** What is involved in the treatment of Wilms' tumor?

    a. _____

    b. _____

    c. _____

(694) **23.** What precaution is taken in a child with a Wilms' tumor to prevent spread of the disease?

    _____

    _____

Answer as either true (T) or false (F).

(697) **24.** Cryptorchidism can affect the development of secondary sex characteristics. _____

(697) **25.** Cryptorchidism increases the risk of testicular cancer in adulthood. _____

THINKING CRITICALLY

1. A child you are caring for is in renal failure. She is being evaluated for a kidney transplant. Use the library to research this topic. Include in your information the selection process, procedure, risks, expense, recovery, and maintenance.

CASE STUDY

1. Three-year-old Tucker is hospitalized with nephrotic syndrome. Tucker is pale, lethargic, anorexic, and has generalized edema.
    a. Tucker is put on steroid therapy. What are three nursing interventions associated with his treatment?
    b. Plan a menu for Tucker for one day using the nutritional requirements necessary for his recovery.
    c. Tucker likes to lie on his stomach. When you change his position, he is irritable and his mother objects. What would you tell his mother?

Student Name_____

APPLYING KNOWLEDGE

1. While in the clinical area, collect a urine specimen from an infant and a toddler.

2. Measure abdominal girth on a child with ascites.

3. Keep an intake and output record on a child with kidney disease.

4. Use Figure 28-1 in the textbook to label the following.

    a. kidney
    b. ureter
    c. urinary bladder
    d. urethra

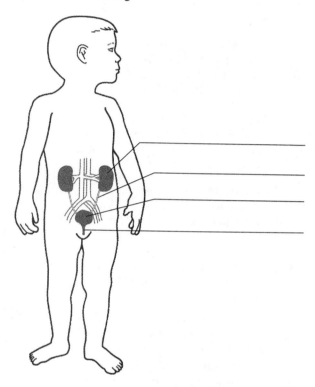

REVIEW QUESTIONS

(690)   1. The treatment of choice for nephrotic syndrome is

1. diuretics.   2. antibiotics.
3. analgesics.   4. steroids.

(690)   2. The child with nephrotic syndrome is at risk for developing

1. skin breakdown.
2. an antigen–antibody reaction.
3. pathologic fractures.
4. urinary stasis.

(684)   3. Which statement about hypospadias is correct?

1. This defect must be corrected in the first few days of life.
2. Fertility will most likely be reduced.
3. The hypospadias may resolve by the first birthday.
4. Surgical repair is usually performed by age 18 months.

(693)   4. What activity restrictions are placed on the child with acute glomerulonephritis?

1. none
2. bed rest for 2 weeks
3. limited until gross hematuria subsides
4. limited for 2 weeks

(694)   5.   Children with acute glomerulonephritis can develop

1.   chronic urinary stasis.
2.   petechiae.
3.   hypotension.
4.   hypertension.

(694)   6.   Wilms' tumors are often discovered
when

1.   children enter school.
2.   the child has flank pain.
3.   blood is noted in the urine.
4.   a routine physical is given.

(687)   7.   Which of the following terms
describes a urethral opening that is
located on the undersurface of the
penis?

1.   hydrocele
2.   phimosis
3.   hypospadias
4.   epispadias

(691)   8.   The risk of urinary tract infections
in girls can be lessened by teaching
them to

1.   wear nylon underwear.
2.   void only when their bladder is
full.
3.   limit fluids after 8:00 PM.
4.   wipe themselves from the front to
the back.

(693)   9.   Acute glomerulonephritis is
thought to be a(n)

1.   antigen–antibody reaction.
2.   autoimmune disease.
3.   primary disease.
4.   infectious disease.

(693)   10.   The urine in acute glomerulonephritis can be described as

1.   straw-colored.
2.   smoky brown.
3.   cloudy and concentrated.
4.   yellow with many mucous shreds.

(689)   11.   A sign of urinary infection in a 6-
year-old is

1.   proteinuria.
2.   perineal rash.
3.   hematuria.
4.   pain during micturition.

(689)   12.   You are caring for a child who has a
ureterostomy. You can expect

1.   urine to be drained from the pelvis
of the kidney.
2.   an opening into the bladder
between the umbilicus and pubis.
3.   surgical implantation of ureters to
outside the abdominal wall.
4.   a tube above the pubis into the bladder to provide urinary drainage.

(693)   13.   Children receiving steroids should

1.   be placed on antibiotics before
there are signs of an infection.
2.   be isolated.
3.   be watched closely for signs of
infection.
4.   taken off the medication after 1
week.

(692)   14.   When weighing diapers on a gram
scale, the conversion from grams to
milliliters is

1.   1 g = 2.5 ml.
2.   1 g = 1 ml.
3.   1 g = 0.5 ml.
4.   1 g = 0.25 ml.

(693)   15.   While the child with nephrotic
syndrome is being treated, he or
she should not receive

1.   antihistamines.
2.   immunizations.
3.   diuretics.
4.   analgesics.

(694)   16.   While caring for a child with
glomerulonephritis, the nurse
observes a rise in the child's blood
pressure. The nurse should

1.   document the change.
2.   document and recheck the blood
pressure in 2 hours.
3.   notify the physician.
4.   withhold fluids until the physician
can visit.

Student Name_____

CROSSWORD PUZZLE

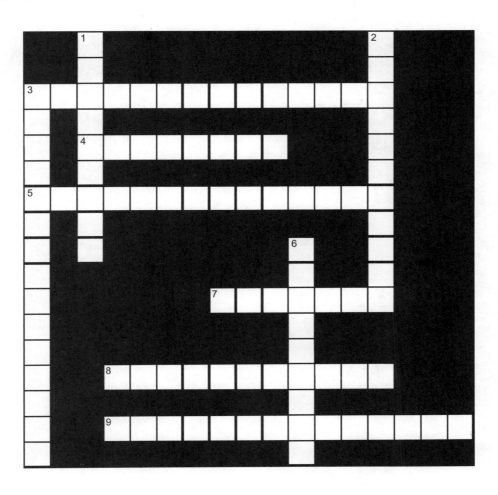

Across

(688) **3.** Distention of the renal pelvis caused by obstruction

(686) **4.** Decreased urinary output

(688) **5.** Infection of the kidney and renal pelvis

(686) **7.** Urge to void but inability to do so

(690) **8.** Absolute neutrophil count below 1000 cells mm^3

(697) **9.** Undescended testicle

Down

(694) **1.** Excessive amount of fluid in the sac that surrounds the testicle

(689) **2.** Surgical opening into the bladder between the umbilicus and pubis

(690) **3.** Decreased level of protein in the blood

(686) **6.** Abnormal number of voidings in a short period

CHAPTER 29

Student Name _____

The Child with a Skin Condition

Answer Key: Textbook page references are provided as a guide for answering these questions. A complete answer key was provided for your instructor.

LEARNING ACTIVITIES

1. Match the terms in the left column with their definitions on the right (a–j).

(719)	_____ autograft	a. benign hemangioma that disappears without treatment
(705)	_____ comedone	b. graft tissue from a source other than human
(717)	_____ debridement	c. removal of dried crusts
		d. graft tissue from cadavers
(702)	_____ exanthem	e. graft tissue from another part of one's body
(718)	_____ heterograft	f. plug of keratin, sebum, and bacteria
		g. skin rash
(718)	_____ homograft	h. graft from the patient's identical twin
		i. infestation of humans by lice
(719)	_____ isograft	j. flat rash (freckles)
(702)	_____ macule	
(712)	_____ pediculosis	
(703)	_____ strawberry nevus	

(700-701) **2.** Describe vernix caseosa.

_____

_____

(701) **3.** What is the purpose of vernix caseosa?

_____

_____

(701)   **4.**   Name three tests used in diagnosing skin conditions.

       a. _____

       b. _____

       c. _____

(701-702) **5.**   Name three of the possible characteristics of skin lesions.

       a. _____

       b. _____

       c. _____

(703)   **6.**   How can the nurse support the parents of a child with strawberry nevus?

       _____

       _____

       _____

(703)   **7.**   What is miliaria?

       _____

(704)   **8.**   How would the nurse advise parents about the treatment for an infant who has seborrheic dermatitis?

       _____

       _____

       _____

(704)   **9.**   How can diaper dermatitis be prevented?

       _____

       _____

(704)   **10.** Briefly describe the pathology of acne.

       _____

       _____

(706)   **11.** Patients taking vitamin A should avoid _____.

Student Name _____

(706) **12.** The main concern of anyone taking Accutane is to

_____.

(706) **13.** A medication that may reduce viral shedding and hasten healing of herpes simplex type 1

infection is _____.

(707) **14.** Eczema is indicative of _____.

(707) **15.** Allergens enter the body of the child with eczema through:

a. _____

b. _____

c. _____

d. _____

(707) **16.** Describe the application of ointment to the skin of a child with eczema.

_____

_____

_____

(710) **17.** The organism responsible for causing scaled skin syndrome is _____.

(711) **18.** What is impetigo and how can it be prevented?

_____

_____

_____

(711) **19.** Describe the treatment of impetigo.

_____

_____

_____

(711-712) **20.** Identify the body parts affected in the following tinea infections.

   a.   Tinea capitis: _____

   b.   Tinea corporis: _____

   c.   Tinea pedis: _____

   d.   Tinea cruris: _____

(711)   **21.** Describe the treatment of tinea capitis.

   _____

   _____

   _____

Answer as either true (T) or false (F).

(711)   **22.** Tinea occurs when fungus invades the hair, the stratum corneum layer of the skin, or the nails. _____

(711)   **23.** Tinea infections are not contagious to others. _____

(711)   **24.** Tinea infections heal more quickly if the affected area is kept warm and moist. _____

(712)   **25.** Name the types and locations of the three kinds of pediculosis.

   a.   _____

   b.   _____

   c.   _____

(713)   **26.** What are scabies?

   _____

   _____

(713)   **27.** List the four types of burns.

   a.   _____

   b.   _____

   c.   _____

   d.   _____

Student Name _____

(713) **28.** When a child is burned by fire near the face, assessing for _____

and _____ is a priority.

(713) **29.** The severity of a burn depends on the _____, _____,

and _____ of involvement.

30. Match the burn classification with the correct description (a–c).

(715) _____ first degree

(715) _____ second degree

(715) _____ third degree

a.   blistered, moist, pink, or red; painful
b.   tough, leathery, dry; painless to touch
c.   skin red but blanches easily and refills quickly; painful

(717) **31.** Indications of an inhalation problem in a patient who has been burned include:

a. _____

b. _____

c. _____

d. _____

(717) **32.** If eschar from burns on the trunk inhibits respirations, an _____ is made in order to prevent restriction of chest movement.

(717) **33.** Urine output is observed _____ in a burn patient.

(717) **34.** What is the rationale for inserting a nasogastric tube into a burn patient?

_____

_____

(717) **35.** Describe how a burn wound is dressed.

_____

_____

_____

_____

_____

(719)   **36.** Describe how protective isolation is instituted with a burn patient.

_____

_____

_____

_____

_____

(719)   **37.** List the signs and symptoms of infection in a burn patient.

a. _____

b. _____

c. _____

d. _____

e. _____

(720)   **38.** What type of diet should a burn patient be given?

_____

_____

_____

(720)   **39.** Analgesics are administered _____ painful procedures, such as dressing changes.

(720-721) **40.** The school nurse is talking with children about preventing frostbite. What should be included in the nurse's explanation about dressing for outdoor activities?

_____

_____

THINKING CRITICALLY

1. Use the nursing process to prepare care for a 9-year-old child who was admitted to the hospital with full-thickness burns of the chest and arms 2 days ago. He is burned over 15% of his body. His treatment plan includes an IV, reverse isolation, occlusive dressings with Silvadene to the wound, regular diet with high-protein feedings between meals, and morphine for pain. What do you consider to be the four most important nursing diagnoses? State expected outcomes of care and nursing interventions for one nursing diagnosis. Compare your care plan with others.

Student Name _____

CASE STUDIES

1. Stacey, a 17-year-old teenager diagnosed with acne vulgaris, is prescribed Accutane because other medications have not been effective.
    a. What can the nurse tell Stacey about the side effects of Accutane?
    b. Stacey asks if there is anything she can do with her diet to improve the acne. What should the nurse tell her?
    c. What are some topical preparations that could be recommended for Stacey's acne?

2. Ten-month-old Taylor is admitted to the hospital with a diagnosis of atopic dermatitis. His face, arms, and legs are erythematous and are covered with vesicles, some of which have crusted over. The physician's orders are Isomil formula, continuous wet compresses of Burrow's solution to extremities, cut fingernails, and place in private room.
    a. What is infantile eczema (atopic dermatitis)?
    b. What does the order for Isomil have to do with Taylor's diagnosis?
    c. Describe how the nurse will prepare the wet compresses, their purpose, documentation, and any special care that will be taken while they are on Taylor.
    d. What are some of the psychologic needs of a child with eczema?
    e. Taylor is irritable and continually attempts to scratch his arms and legs. What can the nurse do to soothe him?

APPLYING KNOWLEDGE

1. When you are in the clinical setting, read the charts and find a description of skin on:
    a. an admission assessment.
    b. a child with a skin disorder.
    c. a child with a burn.

REVIEW QUESTIONS

(706-707) **1.** Which of the following skin conditions is *not* contagious?

1. impetigo
2. *Staphylococcus aureus* infection
3. infantile eczema
4. pediculosis

(712) **2.** Treatment of pediculosis capitis includes

1. treatment of all family members.
2. washing the hair with hydrogen peroxide.
3. laundering clothing and bedding in hot water.
4. cutting the hair of all infested children.

(715) **3.** First-aid treatment of a partial-thickness burn should include

1. application of butter.
2. immersion in cold water.
3. elevation of the involved area.
4. breaking the blisters.

(718) **4.** A full-thickness burn can best be described as

1. red with good refill, painful.
2. mottled, red, dull white, painful.
3. blistered, pink or red, painful.
4. tough, leathery, painless to touch.

(719) **5.** An early sign of sepsis in a burn patient is

1. decreased pulse.
2. erythema.
3. elevated temperature.
4. decreased blood pressure.

(717) **6.** A burn patient with cyanosis and charred lips may need a(n)

1. nasogastric tube.
2. endotracheal tube.
3. Foley catheter.
4. throat culture.

(713) **7.** The priority goal in the management of a severe burn is

1. wound debridement.
2. pain control.
3. fluid replacement.
4. airway maintenance.

(711) **8.** A complication of impetigo is

1. rheumatoid arthritis.
2. nephritis.
3. endocarditis.
4. otitis media.

(706) **9.** Adolescents on Accutane must

1. increase their fluid intake.
2. avoid milk products.
3. avoid pregnancy.
4. avoid strenuous exercise.

(712) **10.** When inspecting children for pediculosis capitis, special attention should be paid to the

1. pubic area.
2. hairline at the back of the neck.
3. area around the forehead.
4. underarms.

(707) **11.** A common manifestation of an allergy in a neonate is

1. port wine stain.
2. eczema
3. strawberry nevus.
4. Mongolian spots.

(706) **12.** Adolescents with acne should be instructed to

1. restrict themselves from chocolate and peanuts.
2. wash their faces at least four times a day.
3. get adequate rest and eat a well-balanced diet.
4. avoid sunshine even if they are not on medication.

(708) **13.** Treatment for eczema includes

1. not holding the infant.
2. hot, steaming baths.
3. dressing the infant warmly.
4. having wet compresses applied.

(720) **14.** A priority in changing the dressing of a burn patient is

1. asking the parents to leave the room.
2. medicating for pain prior to the procedure.
3. limiting the number of dressing changes.
4. doing the procedure in the child's room.

(720) **15.** A child who has been burned eats only a small amount of the food on her tray. The nurse should

1. request an order to start an IV.
2. insert a nasogastric tube for feeding.
3. offer the child small, frequent feedings.
4. leave the tray at the bedside longer.

(713) **16.** Scabies are characterized by

1. round, dry patches on the arms.
2. intense itching.
3. a purulent drainage.
4. round lesions similar to chickenpox.

CHAPTER

30

The Child with a Metabolic Condition

Answer Key: Textbook page references are provided as a guide for answering these questions. A complete answer key was provided for your instructor.

LEARNING ACTIVITIES

1. Match the terms in the left column with their definitions on the right (a–g).

(728) _____ glycosuria

(723) _____ hormones

(728) _____ hyperglycemia

(735) _____ hypoglycemia

(729) _____ Kussmaul respirations

(728) _____ polydipsia

(728) _____ polyphagia

a. excessive thirst
b. constant hunger
c. increased glucose in the blood
d. glucose in the urine
e. type of respirations seen in diabetic acidosis
f. decreased glucose in the blood
g. chemical substances produced by glands

(724) **2.** Tay-Sachs disease is genetically transmitted as a(n) _____

_____ trait.

(725) **3.** _____ and _____

counseling have markedly decreased the occurrence of Tay-Sachs disease.

(725) **4.** List five manifestations of hypothyroidism.

a. _____

b. _____

c. _____

d. _____

e. _____

(725)   **5.**   What is essential to prevent sequelae associated with congenital hypothyroidism?

_____

(725-726) **6.**   Describe the pathophysiology of diabetes insipidus.

_____

(726)   **7.**   The initial signs of diabetes insipidus are _____

and _____.

(726-727) **8.**   What would the nurse teach parents about administering DDAVP nasal spray to a child with diabetes insipidus?

_____

(727)   **9.**   Describe the pathophysiology of diabetes mellitus.

_____

_____

_____

_____

(727)   **10.**   Diabetes mellitus is considered to be a(n) _____ disease.

(727)   **11.**   Children usually have type _____ diabetes mellitus. This means there is a(n)

_____ deficiency of insulin.

(728)   **12.**   The onset of type 1 insulin-dependent diabetes is increased in pubescent children. Give two possible causes of this increase.

a.   _____

_____

b.   _____

_____

(728)   **13.**   What are the three "Ps" of type I (insulin-dependent) diabetes mellitus?

a.   _____

b.   _____

c.   _____

Student Name _____

(728) **14.** What is the most reliable test to diagnose diabetes mellitus?

_____

(728) **15.** What test measures glycemic levels over a period of months?

_____

(729) **16.** List the three goals of treatment in type I diabetes mellitus.

a. _____

b. _____

c. _____

(730) **17.** Children with diabetes have problems associated with their stage of growth and development. Give at least one example of a problem for each age group.

a. Infant _____

b. Toddler _____

c. Preschool child _____

_____

d. School-age child _____

_____

e. Adolescent _____

(732) **18.** List three goals of nutritional management for the child with type I diabetes mellitus.

a. _____

_____

b. _____

_____

c. _____

_____

(733) **19.** The standard form of insulin is _____.

(734)   **20.**   Describe insulin injection site rotation.

_____

_____

_____

_____

_____

(735)   **21.**   List three reasons why a child might go into insulin shock.

a.   _____

b.   _____

c.   _____

(736)   **22.**   What is the immediate treatment of a child suspected of having an insulin reaction?

_____

_____

(736)   **23.**   _____ may be given for the
treatment of severe hypoglycemia.

(736)   **24.**   Explain the Somogyi phenomenon.

_____

_____

_____

(737)   **25.**   List three precautions in the foot care of a child with diabetes.

a.   _____

b.   _____

_____

c.   _____

_____

Student Name_____

(737) **26.** When a child with diabetes plans to travel, what should be done prior to and during the trip?

a. _____

b. _____

c. _____

d. _____

27. Match each sign or symptom with its cause. (Causes may be used more than once.)

(729)   _____ fruity breath

(729)   _____ headache

(729)   _____ diaphoretic

(729)   _____ abdominal pain

(729)   _____ tremors

(729)   _____ deep, rapid respirations

a. hypoglycemia
b. hyperglycemia

Answer as either true (T) or false (F).

(727)   **28.** The symptoms of diabetes mellitus appear more slowly in children. _____

(724)   **29.** Growth hormone should be administered at bedtime. _____

(727)   **30.** Water intake should be limited for the child with diabetes insipidus. _____

(732)   **31.** Children with type I diabetes mellitus require special foods. _____

(737)   **32.** The child with type I diabetes mellitus is able to participate in almost all sports activities. _____

(725)   **33.** If left untreated, congenital hypothyroidism can result in mental retardation. _____

THINKING CRITICALLY

1. Plot a curve showing the peaks and duration of action for a child who is receiving a combination of regular and NPH insulin at 7:30 AM and 5:30 PM.

CASE STUDY

1. Anne, a 16 years old, is newly diagnosed with type I diabetes mellitus. She is a cheerleader and plays basketball. Since her diagnosis, Anne's parents are constantly with Anne and are very protective of her.
   a. Anne is placed on a constant carbohydrate diet. What should the nurse tell her about the advantages of this type of diet?
   b. Anne asks if she can still play basketball and remain a cheerleader. What should the nurse tell her about these activities?
   c. Anne becomes very impatient with her mother and accuses her of hovering. How can emotional turmoil have an effect on adolescent with diabetes?

APPLYING KNOWLEDGE

1. While in the clinical area, teach a child or a parent to give insulin.

2. While in the clinical area, teach a family home glucose monitoring.

3. Care for a child in diabetic ketoacidosis.

REVIEW QUESTIONS

(735) 1. A child receives Lispro insulin before breakfast. She should eat her meal
1. immediately.
2. within 15 minutes.
3. within 40 minutes.
4. within 60 minutes.

(734) 2. Children can usually give their own insulin injections after the age of
1. 7 years.   2. 9 years.
3. 11 years.   4. 13 years.

(726) 3. An initial sign of diabetes insipidus is
1. polyphagia.
2. polydipsia.
3. excessive perspiration.
4. hyperglycemia.

(736) 4. To treat a child having an insulin reaction, the nurse should give
1. orange juice.
2. unsalted crackers.
3. tea.
4. an apple.

(729) 5. A sign of diabetic ketoacidosis is
1. cold perspiration.
2. decreased heart rate.
3. deep, rapid respirations.
4. slurred speech.

(733) 6. The most common concentration of insulin is
1. U-35 insulin.
2. U-40 insulin.
3. U-80 insulin.
4. U-100 insulin.

Student Name _____

(735) **7.** A type of intermediate-acting insulin is

1. regular insulin.
2. Lente insulin.
3. PZI insulin.
4. Ultralente insulin.

(735) **8.** A frequent cause of hypoglycemia in children is

1. not enough food.
2. too much insulin.
3. illness.
4. poorly planned exercise.

(735) **9.** One sign of an insulin reaction is

1. dry skin.
2. flushed face.
3. cold perspiration.
4. increased thirst.

(735) **10.** Regular insulin is considered to be a(n)

1. rapid-acting insulin.
2. intermediate-acting insulin.
3. long-acting insulin.

(733) **11.** A characteristic common to type I diabetes mellitus is that it

1. is more common in preschool-age children.
2. is often seen in obese individuals.
3. always requires insulin.
4. has few blood sugar fluctuations.

(724-725) **12.** One characteristic of Tay-Sachs disease is

1 diagnosis at birth.
2. there is no cure.
3. increased cure rate if diagnosed before age 6 months.
4. normal growth and development.

(737) **13.** The nurse would teach a child with type I diabetes mellitus to check urine for acetone when he

1. is exercising.
2. is ill.
3. has eaten a high-carbohydrate diet.
4. is going through a growth spurt.

(725) **14.** Screening infants for hypothyroidism is

1. ordered for children of high-risk families.
2. done on all infants at 6 months of age.
3. done on all infants at birth.
4. ineffective.

(725) **15.** Thyroid hormone replacement for children with hypothyroidism

1. can be discontinued after the child has gone through puberty.
2. is lifelong.
3. is gradually discontinued after the child can eat solids.
4. is started after the infant is weaned.

31 The Child with a Communicable Disease

Answer Key: Textbook page references are provided as a guide for answering these questions. A complete answer key was provided for your instructor.

LEARNING ACTIVITIES

1. Match the terms in the left column with their definitions on the right (a–f).

(747) _____ epidemic

(749) _____ erythema

(747) _____ fomite

(747) _____ prodromal period

(747) _____ vector

(750) _____ vesicle

a. interval between the earliest symptoms and the appearance of the rash or fever

b. inanimate material that absorbs and transmits infection

c. insect or animal that carries and spreads a disease

d. sudden increase of a communicable disease in a localized area

e. diffused, reddened area on the skin

f. circular, reddened area on the skin that is elevated and contains fluid

(747-748) **2.** List three factors related to host resistance to disease.

a. _____

b. _____

c. _____

(748) **3.** What is an opportunistic infection?

_____

_____

(748) **4.** A child developed a wound infection while he was hospitalized postoperatively. This is called

a _____ infection.

(748)   **5.**   Vaccines provide _____ _____ immunity to disease.

(748)   **6.**   A child received tetanus serum to prevent lockjaw. This is an example of _____ immunity.

(749)   **7.**   The Center for Disease Control recommends _____ precautions for all patients. This involves _____ and

_____ .

(749)   **8.**   When would the nurse use contact precautions?

_____

(749)   **9.**   Describe the components of protective isolation.

_____

10.   Match the following terms with the correct description (a–e).

(749)   _____ macule

(750)   _____ papule

(750)   _____ vesicle

(750)   _____ pustule

(750)   _____ scab

a.   dried pustule covered with a crust
b.   circular, reddened area on the skin that is elevated and contains fluid
c.   circular, reddened area on the skin
d.   circular, reddened area on the skin that is elevated and contains pus
e.   circular, reddened area on the skin that is elevated

(751)   **11.**   List six contraindications to administration of a live virus vaccine.

a.   _____

b.   _____

c.   _____

d.   _____

e.   _____

f.   _____

(742)   **12.**   The incubation period for varicella is _____ .

(742)   **13.**   How long is the child with varicella contagious? _____

Student Name_____

(743)   **14.** Describe the appearance of the child with fifth disease.

_____

(744)   **15.** List the manifestations of infectious mononucleosis.

    a. _____

    b. _____

    c. _____

    d. _____

(744)   **16.** Nursing interventions related to the care of a child with hepatitis A include:

    a. _____

    b. _____

    c. _____

    d. _____

(745)   **17.** Lyme disease is spread by _____.

(745)   **18.** Identify three actions that can be taken to prevent Lyme disease.

    a. _____

    b. _____

    c. _____

(756)   **19.** List the three ways in which children can acquire the human immunodeficiency virus (HIV).

    a. _____

    b. _____

    c. _____

(756-759) **20.** Identify three nursing diagnoses for a toddler with AIDS.

    a. _____

    b. _____

    c. _____

THINKING CRITICALLY

1. Four-month-old Orlando has come to the pediatrician's office for his well-child checkup. His mother tells you that Orlando's immunizations are up to date. Refer to the immunization schedule (Figure 31-6) to determine which immunizations he should receive at this visit.

2. You are asked to care for an adolescent with pelvic inflammatory disease. You know that she has been sexually active and has a history of STDs. Think about this situation and then write down your thoughts about this patient.

3. Develop a plan to teach adolescents about the prevention of sexually transmitted diseases.

APPLYING KNOWLEDGE

1. Contact your local health department for information about educating the public about STDs. Request pamphlets and other written materials.

2. Assist nurses in a public health clinic to administer immunizations.

REVIEW QUESTIONS

(752) 1. Which of the following diseases does not require a routine immunization?

   1. chickenpox
   2. smallpox
   3. measles
   4. German measles

(747) 2. The period that refers to the initial stage of a disease between the earliest symptoms and the appearance of the rash or fever is the

   1. incubation period.
   2. infectious period.
   3. prodromal period.
   4. stage one period.

(748) 3. An infection acquired in a health-care facility during hospitalization is termed a(n)

   1. opportunistic infection.
   2. nosocomial infection.
   3. acquired infection.
   4. natural infection.

(749) 4. Patients with tuberculosis, varicella, and rubeola would require which type of infection precautions?

   1. large droplet infection precautions
   2. airborne infection precautions
   3. communicable disease precautions
   4. indirect transmission precautions

(750) 5. A circular, reddened area on the skin that is elevated and contains fluid is a

   1. vesicle.   2. pustule.
   3. macule.   4. papule.

(742) 6. The incubation period for chickenpox is

   1. 1–2 weeks.   2. 2–3 weeks.
   3. 3–4 weeks.   4. 4–5 weeks.

Student Name_____

(749) **7.** A child with pertussis would be placed in which type of isolation?

1. large droplet infection precautions
2. airborne infection precautions
3. communicable disease precautions
4. protective isolation precautions

(749) **8.** The most important nursing action in preventing the spread of infection is

1. the administration of antibiotics.
2. placing all children in private rooms.
3. good hand washing.
4. good nutrition.

(743) **9.** Koplik's spots in the mouth can be found in

1. chickenpox.
2. rubella.
3. rubeola.
4. mumps.

(742) **10.** The risk of secondary infection in communicable diseases is reduced by

1. giving all children antibiotics.
2. keeping fingernails short.
3. forcing fluids.
4. isolating the child.

(743) **11.** The disease that causes a "slapped cheek" appearance is

1. Lyme disease.
2. roseola.
3. strep throat.
4. fifth disease.

(742) **12.** Chickenpox can be life-threatening to a child who

1. is under 6 months of age.
2. is immunocompromised.
3. runs a high fever.
4. contracts the disease a second time.

(752) **13.** A child should receive the measles, mumps, rubella (MMR) vaccine at

1. 4 months.   2. 6 months.
3. 15 months.   4. 24 months.

(753) **14.** If a vaccination series is interrupted,

1. the series must start over.
2. it continues without restarting the entire series.
3. the age of the child determines if the series must be restarted.
4. the child must wait 6 months before restarting the series.

CHAPTER 32

The Child with an Emotional or Behavioral Condition

Answer Key: Textbook page references are provided as a guide for answering these questions. A complete answer key was provided for your instructor.

LEARNING ACTIVITIES

1. Match the terms in the left column with their definitions on the right (a–f).

(767)	_____ gateway substances	a. thoughts about suicide
(762)	_____ milieu therapy	b. attempt at a suicidal-type action that does not result in injury
(762)	_____ psychosomatic	c. action that is seriously intended to cause death
(764)	_____ suicidal attempt	d. physical and social environment
(764)	_____ suicidal gestures	e. common household products that can be abused to achieve an altered state of consciousness
(764)	_____ suicidal ideation	f. bodily dysfunctions that seem to have emotional and organic bases

(762) 2. Identify three interventions that may be used in the treatment of emotional or behavioral conditions.

a. _____

b. _____

c. _____

(762) 3. Creating an _____ _____ environment is basic to all forms of therapy.

(762) 4. List four psychological disturbances seen in children who come from dysfunctional families.

a. _____

b. _____

c. _____

d. _____

(763)   **5.**   List three signs of autism usually seen by 1 year of age.

     a. _____

     b. _____

     c. _____

(763)   **6.**   Describe the treatment of autism.

     _____

     _____

     _____

(763)   **7.**   What strategies can the nurse use when caring for a child with autism during hospitalization?

     _____

(764)   **8.**   Describe the nurse's role in caring for a child with obsessive-compulsive disorder.

     _____

(764)   **9.**   List five common signs and symptoms experienced by adolescents who are depressed.

     a. _____

     b. _____

     c. _____

     d. _____

     e. _____

(764)   **10.**   Manifestations of suicidal behavior include:

     a. _____

     b. _____

     c. _____

     d. _____

     e. _____

     f. _____

Student Name_____

(764)   **11.** Give an example of a question the nurse might ask an adolescent suspected of being suicidal.

_____

_____

(767)   **12.** State the four levels of substance abuse.

a. _____

b. _____

c. _____

d. _____

(767)   **13.** What are the two types of drug dependence?

a. _____

b. _____

(767, 769) **14.** List two strategies for the prevention of substance abuse.

a. _____

_____

b. _____

_____

(769-770) **15.** What are the four predominant coping patterns of children of alcoholics?

a. _____

b. _____

c. _____

d. _____

(771)   **16.** Give two examples of each of the following clinical manifestations of a child with attention deficit hyperactivity disorder (ADHD).

a. Inattention _____

_____

b. Impulsiveness _____

_____

c.   Hyperactivity _____

_____

(771)   **17.**   Describe the treatment of ADHD.

_____

_____

(772)   **18.**   The primary symptom of anorexia nervosa is _____.

(772)   **19.**   List five of the possible body changes associated with anorexia nervosa.

a.   _____

b.   _____

c.   _____

d.   _____

e.   _____

(772)   **20.**   List some of the common behaviors of families of children with anorexia nervosa.

_____

_____

(772)   **21.**   Describe the eating habits of a child with bulimia.

_____

(773)   **22.**   Siblings of children with a long-term illness are at risk for developing

_____ and _____.

THINKING CRITICALLY

1.   In what way should care be altered when caring for a child with asthma who is also diagnosed as having ADHD?

Student Name _____

CASE STUDY

1. Nine-year-old Krystof has arrived at the same-day surgery unit for dental extractions. Krystof was diagnosed with autism when he was 3 years old.
   a. What factors might influence Krystof's reaction to this hospital experience?
   b. You will be admitting Krystof to the unit. What information specific to autism would you elicit from Krystof's mother during the admission process?
   c. His mother tells you that Krystof is very anxious about his surgery. What strategies will you use to interact with Krystof?
   d. After Krystof has been taken to the operating room, his mother says, "I don't understand why my other children seem to resent Krystof." What do you think is the reason for this? How would you respond to this statement?

APPLYING KNOWLEDGE

1. Discuss in class how an adolescent suspected of being suicidal should be interviewed.

2. List two nursing diagnoses associated with depression. Discuss in a group how nursing care should be implemented for these diagnoses.

3. Care for a child who is admitted to the hospital with an emotional disorder.

4. Interview the family members of a child with ADHD. What impact has this condition had on them, individually and as a family?

REVIEW QUESTIONS

(764) 1. The risk of death increases in a suicidal adolescent when
   1. he is an only child.
   2. he has a learning disorder.
   3. he has a definite plan of action.
   4. his parents are divorced.

(768) 2. Alcohol is known to be a
   1. depressant.
   2. high source of protein.
   3. stimulant.
   4. antidepressant.

(768) 3. Marijuana has which of the following physical effects?
   1. bradycardia
   2. increased awareness
   3. anorexia
   4. tachycardia

(769) 4. The street name for a form of cocaine is
   1. crap.   2. smack.
   3. hash.   4. crack.

(767) 5. Primary to prevention of substance abuse in children is a
   1. positive self-image.
   2. strong religious belief.
   3. strict family.
   4. good education.

(769) 6. Adolescents who seek help for a substance abuse problem usually do so because
   1. there are no other options.
   2. they have friends in treatment.
   3. they realize they need help.
   4. their family encourages them.

(765)   7.   If a nurse suspects an adolescent is contemplating suicide, he or she should

1.   avoid the subject.
2.   ask the parents if they agree.
3.   ask the adolescent directly if he or she is thinking of killing him- or herself.
4.   observe him or her closely.

(764)   8.   The best response to a depressed adolescent is

1.   "Cheer up, things will get better."
2.   "Let's talk about how you are feeling."
3.   "Things always seem worse than they are."
4.   "You are so lucky to have so many friends."

(767)   9.   The type of drug dependence that causes withdrawal symptoms is called

1.   psychologic.
2.   pharmacologic.
3.   physical.
4.   mental.

(767)   10. Adolescents who drink even small amounts of alcohol are at increased risk to

1.   develop acne.
2.   become obese.
3.   have a drop in their intelligence.
4.   have an accident.

(772)   11. Bulimia is described as

1.   binge eating followed by self-induced vomiting.
2.   inability to eat due to fear of gaining weight.
3.   a systemic infection caused by a parasite.
4.   a secondary infection caused by a parasite.

(764)   12. A 16-year-old male who has broken off with his girlfriend threatens to kill himself. The nurse knows that this behavior

1.   is attention-seeking.
2.   should be taken seriously.
3.   should be ignored.
4.   is a normal reaction to the situation.

(762)   13. The 5-year-old child of parents who have recently divorced has started sucking her thumb. The nurse knows that this is

1.   a normal growth and development phase of many 5-year-olds.
2.   cause for immediate psychiatric referral.
3.   response to the parent's separation.
4.   probably unrelated to the parent's divorce.

(771)   14. Children with ADHD

1.   may experience low self-esteem.
2.   are usually high achievers.
3.   usually have many friends.
4.   excel when given tasks that require intricate work.

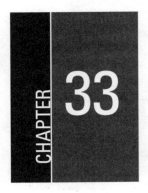

CHAPTER 33

Complementary and Alternative Therapies in Maternity and Pediatric Nursing

Answer Key: Textbook page references are provided as a guide for answering these questions. A complete answer key was provided for your instructor.

LEARNING ACTIVITIES

(775)   **1.**   Give examples of the following therapies. Can you identify examples other than those listed in the text?

     a.   Complementary therapy _____

     _____

     b.   Alternative therapy _____

     _____

(775-777)   **2.**   What is the current status of regulation and licensure in the United States related to complementary and/or alternative therapies?

     _____

     _____

(778)   **3.**   a.   What conditions can massage therapy benefit?

     _____

     b.   What are contraindications for use of massage therapy? Why?

     _____

     _____

(779)   **4.**   What is the use of an acupressure wristband during pregnancy?

     _____

(779)   **5.**   What are cautions and potential risks of homeopathic medicines?

_____

_____

(779-780) **6.**   a.   List some essential oils that should not be used during pregnancy.

_____

_____

b.   List oils that may be beneficial during pregnancy. What are their effects?

_____

_____

c.   List essential oils that may benefit children with chronic pain.

_____

_____

(780)   **7.**   a.   How is guided imagery believed to be therapeutic?

_____

b.   How can a nurse use guided imagery to help a woman in labor?

_____

_____

(781)   **8.**   List two problems in terms of regulation or control that the consumer encounters when using an herbal product.

a.   _____

b.   _____

(781)   **9.**   What are the cautions if herbal remedies are used during pregnancy, breastfeeding, or in children?

a.   Use during pregnancy _____

_____

b.   Use when breastfeeding _____

_____

c.   Use in children _____

_____

Student Name_____

(782)   **10.** List 12 herbs that a pregnant woman should not take.

a. _____

b. _____

c. _____

d. _____

e. _____

f. _____

g. _____

h. _____

i. _____

j. _____

k. _____

(781-782) **11.** Why should a pregnant woman avoid the herbs listed in question 10?

_____

(782, 784) **12.** List four methods used as an alternative to hormone replacement therapy to manage the discomforts of menopause.

a. _____

b. _____

c. _____

d. _____

APPLYING KNOWLEDGE

   1. Choose a complementary or alternative therapy that you have heard of, used, or considered using. Go to the web site for the National Center for Complementary and Alternative Medicine at the National Institutes of Health at http://nccam.nih.gov/. Identify information about the uses, effectiveness, and adverse effects of the therapy you have chosen.

   2. Attend a childbirth class in which preparation for labor is covered. What complementary therapies do you see taught to expectant parents in the class?

REVIEW QUESTIONS

(776-777) **1.** What is the most important reason a nurse should ask specifically about a patient's use of complementary or alternative therapy when admitting him or her to the hospital?

1. Use of these therapies gives insight into the person's cultural background.
2. Most therapies are promoted by those with little education in their use.
3. Knowledge of possible interactions with prescribed traditional drugs reduces the chance of complications.
4. The patient and family should be educated about the harmful effects of most complementary therapies.

(782, 784) **2.** A woman is troubled by discomforts such as hot flashes as she approaches menopause. She prefers to avoid hormone replacement therapy because her mother had breast cancer and she asks the nurse if natural remedies will help her. The best answer by the nurse is that

1. these discomforts are normal for menopause and will gradually go away.
2. some herbs may help her symptoms but she should consult her physician before using them.
3. most herbs are regulated by the Food and Drug Administration as estrogen would be regulated.
4. heat therapy is the most reliable way to reduce nighttime hot flashes.

(778) **3.** A 3-year-old child is hospitalized for pneumonia. The nurse notes marks on the abdomen and asks the parents about how the child received them. The parents reply that they often use "coin rubbing" when the child is ill. Based on this explanation, the nurse should

1. document the marks and the parents' explanation for them.
2. consult with child protective services because of possible abuse.
3. explain to the parents that this practice cannot heal an infection.
4. tell the parents that coin rubbing is dangerous to small children.

(778) **4.** Energy therapy that may relieve nausea and vomiting associated with chemotherapy is

1. effleurage of the abdomen.
2. cold applied to the head.
3. aromatherapy with essential oils and essences.
4. transcutaneous electrical nerve stimulation.

(781) **5.** A woman, 24 weeks gestation, is having her regular antepartal checkup. She tells the nurse that acupressure has helped her with many discomforts, including the nausea she felt during early pregnancy. The best nursing response is

1. pressure on the bottom of her foot can help relieve the backache that often occurs during late pregnancy.
2. acupuncture is safer than acupressure for relief of discomforts that are common during early and late pregnancy.
3. several areas for pressure should be avoided during pregnancy to reduce the risk for preterm birth.
4. it is best to avoid all types of unproven complementary therapies when she is pregnant.

Student Name _____

(781) **6.** When determining the dose of herbal therapy, the practitioner uses the

1. person's body weight.
2. person's age.
3. largest dose the person can tolerate.
4. immune status of the person.

(781) **7.** A woman has taken a number of vitamins and herbal therapies throughout her pregnancy. To avoid infection while she is breastfeeding she takes large quantities of vitamin C. The nurse should advise the woman that

1. vitamin C can reduce the chance of infection in both her and the baby.
2. vitamin C is a fat-soluble vitamin and should not be taken in large doses.
3. taking vitamin C with a milk product will enhance its absorption.
4. colic is more likely in the baby if she takes large amounts of vitamin C.

(784) **8.** A woman who is 30 weeks pregnant enjoys a sauna many times to help her relax after work. The nurse should advise her to

1. keep the heat level low enough to avoid sweating.
2. all heat therapy is contraindicated during pregnancy.
3. she should leave the sauna if her pulse reaches 120.
4. have another person with her when she uses the sauna.

CROSSWORD PUZZLE

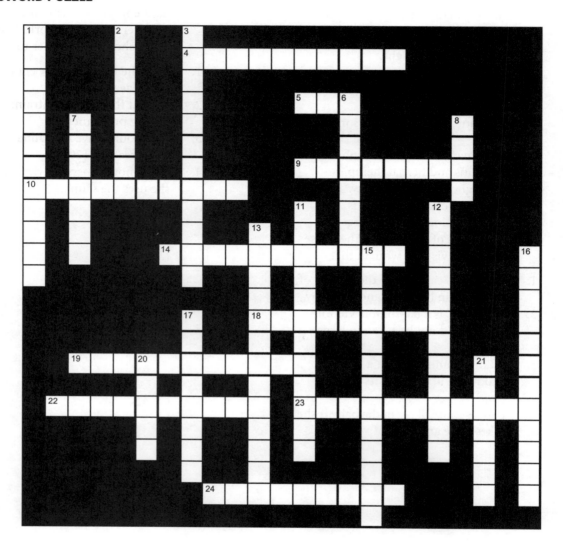

Across

(779) **4.** Use of plants, herbs, and earth minerals to stimulate the body's immune system or help specific health problems

(777) **5.** Abbreviation for the agency that regulates drugs for effectiveness and safety

(778) **9.** Pathway to a specific organ or body part; used in acupuncture and acupressure

(778) **10.** Type of massage used during labor

(780-781) **14.** Use of an electronic instrument to help a person recognize muscle tension

(778) **18.** Practitioner who combines traditional and manipulative therapy

(778-779) **19.** Stimulation of nerve cells using very thin needles

(778) **22.** Another name for traditional medicine

(775) **23.** Unconventional therapy that replaces mainstream therapy

(776) **24.** Mexican cultural folk healer

Student Name_____

Down

(780)   **1.** Therapy delivered by suggestions given to a person when he or she is in a state of induced sleep

(781)   **2.** Digitalis originates in this plant

(781)   **3.** Nerve energy is thought to restore or maintain health; care involves the relationship between the spinal column and nervous system

(779)   **6.** Hindu healing that considers the biological rhythms of nature

(778)   **7.** Pressure, stretching, and manipulation of the fascia to increase muscle and bone function

(778)   **8.** Acronym for transcutaneous electrical nerve stimulator

(780)   **11.** Use of water to promote relaxation

(776)   **12.** Use of many medications

(778)   **13.** Type of massage to relieve muscle tension and trigger points of pain

(775)   **15.** Nontraditional therapy used in conjunction with conventional therapy

(779)   **16.** Use of concentrated essential oils combined with steam or baths to inhale or bathe the skin

(781)   **17.** Form of herbal remedy that contains a large quantity of alcohol

(781)   **20.** Opiates for pain are related to this plant

(779)   **21.** Finger pressure used to prevent disease